The Bounce

The Complete SuperBound® Guidebook
to 21st-Century Rebound Exercise

The Bounce

The Complete SuperBound® Guidebook to 21st-Century Rebound Exercise

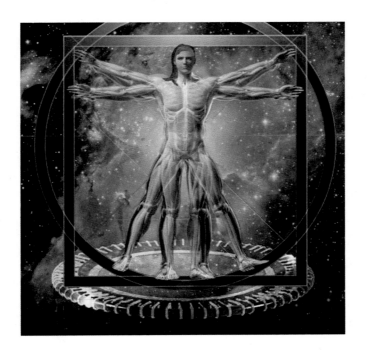

Joy Daniels & Jordan Gruber
Illustrations by Krisztina Lazar

SuperBound LLC
Menlo Park 2020

SuperBound LLC
205 Pope St.
Menlo Park, California, 94025, USA
http://www.superbound.net

ISBN 978-1-7348399-3-7 (print paperback)
ISBN 978-1-7348399-1-3 (print hardback)
ISBN 978-1-7348399-0-6 (ebook)

10 9 8 7 6 5 4 3 2 1

To send correspondence to the authors of this book, please contact the authors directly at info@SuperBound.net

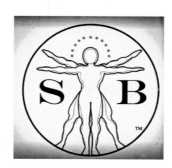

Acknowledgements

We would like to thank many people for their contributions to this volume as well as for their friendship, good humor, and support. This includes all those who took a turn at editing or otherwise improving previous versions of this book, including Krisztina Lazar (whose fabulous illustrations grace these pages), Christopher Allen, Dara Silverman, and David Jon Peckinpaugh. My sister Helene Gruber gets special thanks for her heroic last-second proofreading so we could meet our trademark deadline. And special thanks to our book formatter, Marko Markovic from 5mediadesign, for his excellent work. Additional thanks go to:

Kathy Scally Abrignani, Vern Ader, Lasara Allen, Colleen Meeks Bastys, Boomer, Sheila Brady, Doug Brignole, Marina (Takahashi) Browe, Al Carter, Diana Chambers, Kathleen Daly, Andy Daniels, Carolyn Daniels, Sylvan Daniels, Faye Lewark Daniels, Willow Dea, Gabriel DeWitt, Lena Diethelm, Melissa Dinwiddie, Sylvia Dreiser Farnsworth, Jeremy Edwardes, Bill Eichman, Liz Elms.

Dorothy Fadiman, Jim Fadiman, Esther Gokhale, Marianne Grace, Diana Gruber, Jeramy Hale, Molly Hale, Linda Herreshoff, Tom Howell, Karen Ippolito, Samantha Rae Jackson, Twyla Johnson, Damon Kali, AnnaKarenina Kealoha, Richard Koralek, Ed Lark, Allan Lundell, Morganne Maher, Tom McCook.

Karen McKenzie, Sun McNamee, Vanessa McNeill, Damon Miller, Kelly Angel-ina Munroe, Craig Michael Lie Njie, Amy Hallman Rice, Michelle Robertson, Dr. Carol Robin, Alex Rose, Robert Rudelic, Ken Seeley, Michael Sandler, Ted Selker, Steve Shafarman, Dara Silverman, Gail Slocum, Mitchel Slomiak, Brooke Stapleton, Cynthia Stevenson, Cristiano Verducci, Brian Weller, Jeffry Winters, Phoenix Winters.

We'd also like to thank all those companies—some for decades—that have been manufacturing high quality rebounders and keeping rebound exercise alive. We salute bellicon®, Cellerciser®, JumpSport®, Leaps & Rebounds, Needak®, and ReboundAIR.

Jordan and Joy would each like to thank the members of their families for putting up and down with them. Jordan would also like to thank his cats, as well as the proprietors of every vacation home and hotel where he "secretly" bounced. Joy would like to give a special shout out to her three granddaughters, Ellie, Avi, and Fiya, and her grandson Teague, all of whom have been fascinated with bouncing since the day they were born.

Finally, we would like to acknowledge all of you who, like us, choose to explore and embrace rebound exercise and the Bounce as a profound health and wellness practice.

Medical Advisory and Safety Disclaimer

Rebounding can make you healthier, stronger, illness resistant, toned, and muscular, and can improve your balance, aerobic conditioning, and mood. All of this is possible, in part, because a rebounder is—in more ways than one—a highly leveraged exercise platform. But this means that if you're careless or lose focus, you can hurt yourself. Therefore:

- <u>Don't start a program of rebound exercise without first consulting with your medical care provider.</u>
- <u>Always follow rebounding basic safety rules and guidelines,</u> including:
  - Make sure the equipment is correctly set up and safely used.
  - Make sure you're in a safe physical place and mental state to bounce.
  - Stop bouncing at the first signs of pain or distress. Seek help if your condition doesn't improve within a reasonable amount of time.
  - Continuously supervise all children and pets on or near a rebounder.
- Go slow—and we really do mean S...U...P...E...R   S...L...O...W—when you first start bouncing. Please, don't rush into rebounding only to injure yourself and perhaps never again benefit from the Bounce.
- Always remain conscious and aware, religiously put safety first, and never push past a point of pain or struggle.

The authors and publishers have no formal training or credentials in any medical or fitness area. While this book provides carefully researched and thoughtfully considered information based on published studies, firsthand accounts, and personal experience, it cannot possibly address the unique health history and medical condition of each reader.

We therefore *urge each reader to discuss any new or revised exercise program with their personal healthcare provider*. Rebounding offers a highly customizable exercise platform on which certain techniques and movements may be feasible and useful for some but not other readers. This is *especially true for those with preexisting conditions,* who may require modifying or entirely forgoing having the Bounce in their life. (It can be as simple as a foot problem—severe pronators can be troubled by bungee-based mats—or something as potentially complicated and nuanced as a knee or disc issue.)

Please understand that *we cannot be held responsible for any accidents or injuries that might come about from any individual reader's actions or adaptation of this book's information to his or her own individual circumstances*. Nor can we be held responsible for any accidents, injuries, or mishaps that happen from the use of any rebound exercise equipment. It's your job to keep yourself—and everyone who might come in contact with your rebounder—safe.

Table of Contents

Section I:

An Introduction to the Bounce

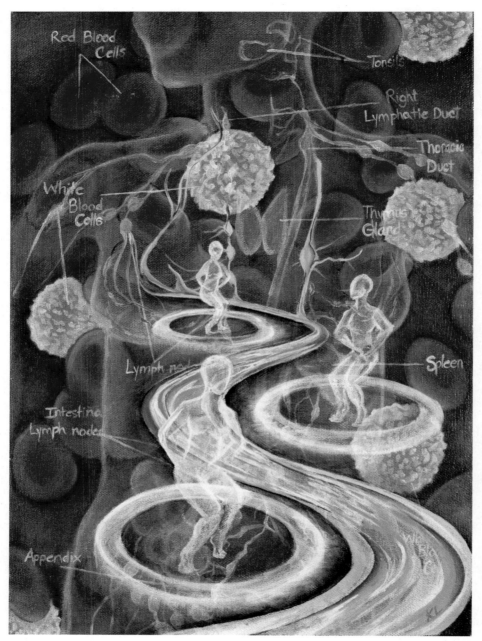

"Lymph Bound" by Krisztina Lazar

Chapter 1:

Fun, Safe, and Highly Effective—
Rebound Exercise Rocks!

Your whole body rises up into the air. For a glorious moment, you're flying!

Like a raptor soaring high amongst the clouds, you're finally breaking free of the grasp of Earth's gravity once and for all!

Until you inevitably reach your peak—after all, "what goes up must come down"—and you feel your entire body rapidly descend toward the rebounder's mat. As the bottoms of your feet first make contact[1] with the mat's pliant surface—or as your center of gravity descends to its lowest point—it feels like you've entered the valley of a roller coaster. The deeper you sink in with all of your weight, the more you slow down, until you reach a magic still point at the very bottom...

a suspended moment of time at the deepest point of the valley, lasting for only the smallest of perceptible moments

1   While many people prefer to be "airborne" at least some of the time, you will still receive many of the benefits of the Bounce even if your toes and heels never completely leave the mat.

...only to be immediately thrown back upward toward the sky! And then, you repeat.

While in that deepest valley, your body—every system and cell, every nerve and muscle fiber, every neuron and proprioceptor—anticipates and prepares for the bounce back up. As the fibers of the mat (powered by springs or elastic bungee bands) lift your body out of the valley and back up again, you're neurologically and experientially propelled toward the sky, toward freedom and enhanced access to all of who you are.

As you soar through the space of 10,000 possibilities, riding and modulating Earth's powerful gravity field, you stimulate and potentiate nearly all of your body's cells, fluids, systems, and structures. And—did we mention?—all of this is usually a ton of fun.

Repeating the cycle, the pressure against your feet feels comforting as you relax into what it feels like to modulate your body in such a natural, pleasurable, and repeatable way. Beginning with the proprioceptive nerve endings in your feet, untold numbers of messages are sent back to your brain, which in turn signals your body to make minuscule muscular adjustments to better maintain your balance, positioning, and momentum.

During each of several dozen bounce cycles that occur over the course of a minute, your core muscles engage, release, and strengthen, and unless you're doing a special sitting, lying, or kneeling movement, your legs fully participate as well. For more of an upper body workout, it's easy (and natural) to add in your arms—which have the double advantage of being immediately available and already weighing a good deal.

Then, on top of that, you can use light handheld weights to get a much more thorough upper body workout. (Rebounding with light handheld weights, as we'll explore in detail later, combines quite a few factors that tone and build muscle.) At the same time, your balance and flexibility are challenged as blood flow and immune system—supporting lymph fluid movement are stimulated. There's a lot that's good for you going on here, all of which we'll unpack for you later. As we hope you'll see, it can be fun, simple, and incredibly beneficial to get going with your own practice of the Bounce.

If only Icarus had had a decent rebounder! He could have experienced flying to the sun—over and over again—becoming stronger and healthier, but not burning out.

Better Than Ever and Definitely *Not* Too Good to Be True!

You've likely seen a rebounder before (although maybe not one quite this cosmic): small and usually circular, with a pliable mat inside a frame, about three to four feet in diameter. Depending on the type and quality of rebounder, the legs raise the frame and mat between eight and fourteen inches off the ground.

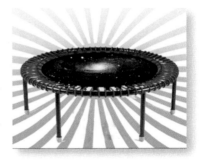

Some of you reading this may even have owned a rebounder with rickety metal springs back in the 80s, when there was a big rebounding fad. Even if you had one, you most likely moved on to other types of exercise long ago—or perhaps you simply became too busy and lost the interest and energy needed to sustain a regular exercise practice. The older we get, the less we tend to move, and few things are better correlated with health and vitality than having regular, diverse, quality movement in your life.

Fortunately, rebound exercise today is far better than it's ever been before. To begin with, today's rebounders are generally far superior to ones from decades ago (and recently there have been some dramatic price breaks on certain types of high-quality models).

Second, as for exactly *how* to bounce, over time it's become quite clear that *there really isn't just one way to bounce.* We see the world of rebound exercise as taking place under a very big tent. However you choose to bounce—your duration, the movements you like to do, the music you listen to or don't listen to, your use or nonuse of handheld weights and other accessories—you will substantially benefit your body, mind, and spirit.

Third, today there are more websites with bouncing classes and routines that you can follow along to than ever before. We encourage you to take a look at these and try out anything that looks good to you. One day soon there may be even more interactive ways to bounce, perhaps along the lines of the Peloton or The Mirror. But having said that, we also strongly encourage you to develop your own day-in and day-out way of bouncing, and to that end, chapter 5 of this book provides a detailed compendium of different ways to bounce, move, use accessories, and more.

We know, we know: it's supposedly so simple, so easy, and so powerfully beneficial in so many ways—from rehabilitation to elite athletic performance, from helping with depression to preventing illness—that it might at first sound too good to be true. But not only have many testified to the verity of these claims (including folks like Bob Hope, Ronald Reagan, Tony Robbins, Madonna, Goldie Hawn, and Gwyneth Paltrow), but it's something you can easily test for yourself. Given how much the price has dropped on a basic, decent-quality bungee-based bouncer, we hope you will.

Our Goals and Intended Audience

> I discovered that exercise actually can be fun! It feels so wonderful to choose to help my body become—and remain—strong. After all, my body's the only forever home I'll always have. I want to enjoy living in it for many years to come.
>
> —Joy Daniels, after two years of rebound exercise practice

Let's take a step back. With rebound exercise—also called "rebounding" or "bouncing"—one person at a time uses a specialized mini-trampoline to move, have fun, and build fitness. Written by two devoted practitioners committed to spreading the transformative qualities of regularly bouncing, this book has two main goals.

Goal # 1: To Illuminate the Benefits and Potential of Rebound Exercise

Our first goal is to calmly and objectively present information about how effective rebounding is, and why it really may be one of the world's best exercises. It's fun, easy, and highly effective; it helps prevent illness and speeds rehabilitation; it's low impact, but you can make it as intense as you like; it builds flexibility, cardio capacity, muscle tone, size, and strength; it has emotional, psychological, and, for some, even spiritual benefits.

Keeping in mind that rebound exercise has been around for about forty years, our intent is to be as comprehensive and up to date as possible.

Goal # 2: To Support You in Trying It for Yourself and Sticking with It

If Goal # 1 is about providing a general comprehensive guide to this fabulous form of movement, exercise, and practice, then Goal # 2 is about helping you give it a go when you're ready to begin or to enhance your current rebound exercise practice.

We not only cover preliminary materials like safety and equipment, but describe exactly how you can begin your own practice, what kinds of movements you can do, and how to put together an effective personal program. We also consider advanced bouncing techniques, movements, and practice protocols. With these two goals in mind, this book is designed as a tool, guide, companion, and objective information source for:

- Those who've never encountered rebounding before;
- Those who used to bounce but gave up on it—whether last week or decades ago;
- Those who have never exercised or haven't exercised regularly for a long time;
- Those who want to move more, feel better, and get sick less;

- Those needing rehabilitative and strengthening work;
- Athletes looking to gain an additional edge;
- Parents looking for fun, safe, and neurologically enhancing activities for kids;
- Baby Boomers looking for increased health and mobility as they age;
- Those seeking psycho-physiological "flow" experiences or ways to embody and enhance their spiritual practice; and
- Those seeking physical, emotional, and even spiritual transformation.

A Health Movement Inspired by Fun-Filled Childhood Memories

Doorway jumpers, bouncing horses, pogo sticks, pogo balls, ball hoppers, moon shoes, inflatable bouncers, bounce houses, diving boards—in one way or another, most of us had access to at least some of these things when we were children. And somehow we instinctively knew how to use them and have fun, as if motion propelled by elastic surfaces was wired into our DNA.

Remember how gravity wasn't such a big deal when we were kids? It was more like a friend and partner than a constant adversary, more something we had fun with than something we had to work against. Now, it seems, we often find ourselves dealing with Ol' Grumpy Gravity, but back then, most of us unconsciously and delightedly challenged and channeled Gee Whiz Gravity whenever we could and in any way we could—by catapulting from the bed or sofa, by jumping from trees, and simply by jumping up and down on the ground as if our very own feet had springs growing out of them.

As kids, you see, our movements weren't restricted to only forward and backward. Our bodies easily maneuvered not just through the well-accustomed horizontal plane, but through the vertical one as well. We had a freedom of movement and motion that strengthened our muscles, lubricated our joints, and kept our ligaments limber. Our 3-D movements and motions constantly worked the proprioceptive mechanisms of our central nervous system, allowing us to infinitely calibrate our body's majestic, multifaceted balancing act and direct exactly where and how we needed to exert force. As we moved without restriction in the vertical plane, we built new neural pathways and taught our bodies how to communicate and function as a whole.

As we get older, most people surrender to gravity as it begins to take its toll on both physical structures and physiological processes. A big part of this is that most people simply stop moving in as wide a variety of ways, planes, and directions. Typically, our lives are spent single-mindedly focused on only one type of movement—forward movement—with our eyes pointing ahead, leading the way. We look straight ahead, walk, bike, and drive forward, and go up and down stairs in one direction. Think of the countless times you've watched someone cross a street without even looking for cars or bikes. And now, with many people literally focused down on their smartphones, it's even worse. Breathing, walking, and other critical functions are compromised by face-down neck-down walking, and our cognitive sovereignty itself may be threatened.

Needless to say, we're not just brains telling the rest of ourselves when to next move our limbs, eat and drink, and use electronic devices. Our brain is inextricably linked to all of who we are, so ignoring or downplaying the mind-body connection inevitably cuts off a large percentage of who we are, including what ultimately makes us human.

The freedom of motion in our bodies—the health of our joints, and the strength and elasticity of our muscles—affects every vital organ in our system, including our brain. The longer and more coherently we move, the better our overall cognitive functioning becomes as our alertness, attention span, concentration, and memory all improve.

The more we relink our minds and bodies, the more our awareness increases, and the more we can be open to everything around us. The more sedentary we become, the more our bodies break down. The amazing Jack LaLanne—fitness guru, early television fitness innovator, and health club pioneer who once performed 1,000 pushups and 1,000 chin-ups in an hour and twenty-two minutes—stated that "The only way you can hurt the body is [to] not use it." Let's now turn to a short summary of the many benefits experienced by those who use rebound exercise as a primary means of moving their bodies.

A Brief Overview of the Benefits of the Bounce

Rebounding's physiological benefits on the body are widely known and for the most part fairly easy to understand. However, I have found nothing that accounts for the euphoric state that washes over me both during and after—sometimes for hours after—my daily bounce. This altered mood almost always ensures a positive outlook throughout my day. I notice it most regularly in my level of confidence—in how happy and proud I am to be who I am, with my body just as it is.

Sometimes before a bounce I fight it, as it's easy to succumb to negative body scrutiny. However, peculiarly, after a bounce something changes in my brain, and I find that I love what I see in the mirror and am 100% more confident in being me, just the way I am, with my own body, just the way it is.

Bouncing helps me be daring and noble. This is a huge bonus and continues to aid me in overcoming and facing societal pressure. We all sometimes feel a need to conform—to look and be a certain way—but I find more of my unique self every time I bounce, and on the odd days when I'm not able to, I miss it sorely in every way. It's fair to say that rebounding has profoundly changed my life.

—Michelle M. Robertson,
Group Rebounding Instructor, Australia

Rebound exercise challenges and leverages gravity in a unique way that can unleash your own healing and transformative potential. It can powerfully exercise your muscles and supportive soft tissue, help heal your body, and stimulate your immune system...all the while providing aerobic conditioning and balance enhancement. It is also fun, can be done at home, and reduces stress while enhancing psychological wellness and even spiritual practice.

Rebounding can work well for and benefit nearly everyone (except those for whom it's contraindicated by an existing medical condition; please see the medical advisory at the beginning of this book). It can increase or improve:

- Strength
- Energy level
- Muscle tone and size
- Cardiovascular fitness
- Balance
- Libido and performance
- Sleep and rest
- Proprioceptive conditioning
- Stamina
- Flexibility
- Relaxation
- Cognitive and emotional clarity
- Spiritual insight
- Skin elasticity and complexion

Given the neurological benefits that follow from training the body to be more coordinated and balanced, it's not surprising that rebound exercise can also increase focus and attention span. We've heard multiple stories of children with attention deficit disorder being able to ride a bike or play the piano much better after they bounce for a while.

Rebound exercise has also been said to help with such conditions as diabetes, osteoarthritis, osteoporosis, edema, neuropathy, vertigo, asthma, back pain, obesity, stress, and even fibromyalgia. We make no specific claims about healing any already existing condition, but instead like to emphasize the odds when considering the long-term benefits of exercising more regularly and effectively. Put simply, if cardio, core strengthening, coordination, balance, or strength training can prevent, rehabilitate, or otherwise benefit a condition, then rebounding may prove a helpful and effective tool.

Rebounding can also be an effective tool for rehabilitation purposes. Its inherently gentle nature—with most of the shock of every bounce cycle being taken by the springs/bungees plus mat combination—is unique.[2] Even in situations where people might initially view themselves as too fragile to bounce, a gentle rebounding practice—perhaps with the use of a stabilizing bar to hold on to at first, or with the person just putting their legs on the rebounder while someone else bounces for them ("buddy bouncing" or assisted bouncing)—can make a world of difference. Remember: even a gentle rocking motion, with your feet not even leaving the mat, will provide many of the benefits of the Bounce.

Again, we realize all of this might seem almost too good to be true. How can something so simple, using what is basically a kind of refined small trampoline, be this beneficial and amazing? How can it possibly be this good for you in so many ways?

The "problem" here, if we want to call it that, is that many people feel that they must work very hard to become healthier or fitter—or to accomplish anything worthwhile, for that matter. So when something is as simple and effective as the Bounce, it tends to get overlooked for the very reason that it seems, well, too simple or childlike. But consider this: don't many of us from time to time already struggle enough with work, life, and other general and unusual circumstances (e.g., our own illness or an illness of someone we love) that make our lives complicated and difficult?

Why not, then, take advantage of something that's very simple and effective? Why not allow yourself to have at least a few minutes a day—every day—that are filled with joy and are good for you on so many levels of your being? We all deserve something special—something simple yet highly effective, and as easy or intense as we want it to be. Something that can truly make a difference! We've found rebounding makes just that difference for us personally, and for many of our friends, and we're eager for it to

---

2   Also worth noting is rebounding's standout ability to rapidly provide whatever increase or decrease of intensity is desired.

make that difference for you too. A journey of a thousand benefits starts with a single step—onto a rebounder—and we're here to guide you every single bounce along the way!

> ### Term of Endearment: Please Use "Rebounder" or "Bouncer," Not "Trampoline"
>
> A quick word about terminology: The exercises and movements discussed in this book are performed on a piece of equipment usually called a "mini-rebounder," a "rebounder," or just a "bouncer." While it's also sometimes called a "trampoline" or "mini-trampoline," we try to discourage this, even if the bouncer is obviously descended from the trampoline.
>
> Trampolines are designed to provide a mostly playful and exciting experience, usually for groups. Rebounders are designed to provide a smooth, safe, and steady personal exercise experience for one person at a time. And while trampolines are designed for stunts—flips, seat drops, etc.—stunts on a rebounder are almost always dangerous and never advised. Yes, they are related types of equipment, but they are also substantially different in their design and everyday usage, and so deserve their different names.
>
> We understand that for those not yet familiar with rebound exercise or the Bounce, the term "mini-trampoline" may be easiest to explain. Still, we would like to request that you shift your language from "trampoline" to "rebounder" or "bouncer." Thanks!

What This Book Will Cover

> Bouncing is amazing! It gives me a renewed confidence
> in my body's ability to transform.
>
> —Ginger Rain

Following this introductory chapter we'll start with a look at "Joy's Journal—The Beginning," detailing her experience of deciding to take on the challenge of establishing a regular bouncing practice for herself. Then in chapter 3 we'll cover the "Major Physical Benefits of the Bounce" in more detail. Chapter 4 is "A Guide to Gear, Safety, and Setting Up"—everything you need to get going.

Chapter 5 is "An Illustrated Compendium of Bounce Types and Movements." Even if you really like online classes (or real-world ones if you have access to them), you'll still want to be able to bounce on your own, so having a compendium or catalog of potential movements and bounce types to try out and experiment with can be very useful. Along the way, we'll discuss adding hand weights to your bouncing sessions. We'll also discuss how to use a rebounder to:

- Rehabilitate injuries;
- De-stress from negative emotions and come back to a grounded center; and
- Perform a bit of rebounder-based yoga, stretching, and related exercise.

Later on, in chapters 6 ("Spiritual/Inner Work Tools and Practices") and 7 ("Joy's Journal: The Sequel, the 45 X 45 Challenge, and Some Q&As"), we'll consider certain metaphysical aspects of the Bounce: the openness felt during times of "flow," the meditative effects of gravity acting on your body, and what exactly it means "to fill in the Vitruvian Sphere" (see box at the end of this chapter). Chapter 8 is "Jordan's Journal—Advanced Protocols and the Limits of Knowledge," where he considers both advanced protocols for bouncing and the limits of knowledge he has run up against (especially his own). Chapter 9 is a short conclusion with some pictures and testimonials from our bouncing friends around the world, along with a few final words of encouragement.

Throughout the book we've incorporated the knowledge, know-how, and profound insights of friends of ours who are bodywork professionals and fitness experts, and who themselves enjoy bouncing. We've also included research information from medical and scientific studies on rebounding—when we can find them and feel they are trustworthy—so you can get a sense of the physiological nuts and bolts of exactly what rebounding can and will do for you.

You'll also read about the experience of many people, just like you, whose journey up and down the path of the Bounce has led to physical benefits and personal growth. We've designed the book as a guidebook, companion, and advocate for your rebounding journey, and hope to foster a worldwide SuperBound rebounding community through real-world and online means. Especially in today's world, where building a strong immune system has never been more important, we want the Bounce to spread as far and wide as possible.

The SuperBound® Approach: What's So "Super" About It?

Rebound exercise is so fun, simple, easy, gentle, and effective that your authors have begun to view it as a kind of super exercise. While there's no evidence (yet!) that regular bouncing will activate your superhuman potential, we feel that "super"—as in "super good," "super fun," and "super effective"—is an entirely appropriate way of looking at it.

The SuperBound project embraces an intentional, "enlightened," and more effective way of performing rebound exercise. A SuperBound practitioner diligently pursues rebound exercise by consciously embracing it as a multidimensional platform for change that enhances (a) many physiological processes, functions, and structures, as well as (b) many of the emotional, mental, and even spiritual dimensions of the human being.

This means, among other things, that the SuperBound approach *directly addresses the inner realities* of bouncing. There are many ways to add an intentional or meditative practice to rebound exercise—or to use it to augment an existing one—or to access and strengthen positive inner states of being. It truly is an integral exercise that seamlessly brings together the outer and the inner, the physical and the psycho-spiritual.

Additionally, since your authors themselves started regularly bouncing (Jordan eighteen years ago, Joy eight years ago), we have personally met or otherwise communicated with people who know a great deal about the human body and mind generally, and about rebounding in particular. A fundamental proposition of the SuperBound approach is that the brilliance and experience of many kinds of teachers—dance and martial arts teachers, experts in meditation and breathwork, specialists in healing, rehabilitation, disabilities, and geriatrics—must all be invited to play, practice, and preach under the big tent that embraces all rebounding activities and knowledge. Wisdom and practical experience from many realms of physical exercise and bodywork can be—and should be—explored and integrated into the wider databank of rebound exercise knowledge.

Yes, there really is no doubt: rebounding is a super exercise—super-fun, super-easy, super-inclusive, and super-effective. Therefore, we decided to go with "SuperBound" as a term for our particular approach to the Bounce, and we even trademarked it.

Congratulations on What's Bound to Be the Coming New You!

Entering the Vitruvian Sphere

As you bounce more frequently, you may find yourself developing an awareness of your body moving in a four-dimensional sphere, space, or bubble that overlays the dimension of time on the three planes or dimensions of movement (up and down, side to side, and back and forth). No single image evokes this experience for us as powerfully as Leonardo da Vinci's famous Vitruvian Man drawing (as paid homage to by the illustration on the cover of this book). Incorporating a vision of this kind of four-dimensional Vitruvian Sphere as you are actually moving through it can be particularly stimulating and healing for your joints, soft tissue, and muscles. We'll say more later about consciously embracing and working within the Vitruvian Sphere.

Every single step of your health and wellness journey up until this moment has led you to this book, to this very page, to these very words.

But no matter how you got here—whether you've never before exercised in your life or you're a fitness enthusiast; whether your doctor recommended that you begin a workout program or you're a high-level athlete looking to further improve; whether you used to rebound back in the day on a big trampoline or a 1980s rebounder with crummy springs; whether you've never even heard of rebounding before now; whether you're in terrific shape or need to tone or gain some muscle and lose some fat; whether you're recovering from an injury, have a chronic condition, or are in perfect health; whether you're relatively old or quite young; and whether you've never heard of rebounding or already regularly practice the Bounce—we are delightedly welcoming you into our rebounding community with open arms.

So, again, welcome! In chapter 3 we'll turn back to a more complete description of the physical benefits of rebound exercise, but for now we invite you to turn the page and start on the first part of Joy's Journal. Here you can follow her eight-week real-time first-person account of beginning the Bounce and developing a regular rebound exercise practice.

Chapter 2:

Joy's Journal—The Beginning

A Question of Balance:
What am I up to, and down for...
And how do I do it?

[This chapter presents the personal journal notes that Joy Daniels kept after Jordan first asked her to consider trying out and committing to a rebounding practice. They have been somewhat modified to make them easier to read and fit into the flow of this book.]

Week 1:
Saying "Yes" to What Might Have Been an Exercise in Futility

The Offer

As my friends will all confirm, I've never had any interest in exercise whatsoever.

So I think it's hilarious that Jordan asked me to be a test case for *anything* to do with an exercise program. Me? I only exercise inadvertently, never on purpose. (OK, I've danced a lot throughout my entire life, but never once considered it "exercise.") His request will surely turn out to have been an exercise (hah hah) in futility.

You see, during my elementary school years I was one of those unpopular kids—small, nonathletic, and shy. (Yes, believe it or not, I was once quite shy.) I was always picked last for every sports team and activity during gym class. The dislike and even aversion I developed toward all things exercise-related has stayed with me my entire life.

Then I thought some more about Jordan's offer. Such an experiment might be good for me, I thought, so sure, why not? I'll just have to prove to myself that I can do it.

The "it" that I've agreed to is to *literally bounce up and down on a "rebounder" or kind of mini-trampoline.* I'll start slowly, then safely but surely build up my stamina. My goal over the next six months will be to reach and maintain a regular rebounding practice for half an hour a day, five out of seven days. That's two and a half hours a week. No big deal, right? We'll just have to see if I like it, and what the results are.

It's Here!

With my long-awaited shipment delivered, my rebounder has finally come home!

This means I'm now a genuine test case.

Or I will be after tonight, since some old friends are coming over for dinner shortly. The big square cardboard box remains unopened throughout the evening. Sitting there, leaning against the back of my front hallway's green velvet couch, it seems to beckon to me. Needing to navigate around it, my dinner guests ask what it is. I tell them I'm involved in an exercise program, and it's my new tool. They laugh, assuming I'm joking.

I wait until the following morning to unpack my shiny new tool and begin. With the end of the cardboard box slit open, I slide out the circular frame of the rebounder. Then I place it on the floor and screw in the shiny silver legs. When I flip the rebounder right side up I have to grin: it looks like a miniature UFO just landed directly in front of me!

It's perfectly round, with bright orange bungee cords attached to a firm but giving mat in the center. I almost expect it to start rotating of its own accord, then rise up into the air and start flying. Ha!

Stepping On and Rocking It (Very Gently)

I feel compelled to anchor this obviously well-crafted circular object to the earth by stepping onto it right away with my bare feet.

At first I just stand quietly in the center, balancing. Jordan has advised me to take things very, very slow. I don't want to rush by seeing how high I can bounce off the mat or how long I can last at full tilt. It's imperative to get a real sense of an instrument such as this before beginning to play it.

Jordan also cautioned me that I might actually feel some vertigo or dizziness the first few times I bounced. "Always be slow and careful when getting on and off the rebounder," he said. "And always be aware of the vast difference between having your feet and body supported by the soft, pliant surface of the rebounder's mat, and how it feels when you land on hard, unforgiving ground."

As it turns out, I'm hugely grateful for the warnings of what to expect. I've never been one to enjoy carnival rides, and sometimes I get extreme vertigo. Whenever I find myself near the edge of a high balcony or a cliff lookout area, I immediately get dizzy. If I went just one step closer... it feels like I'd get sucked right off the edge! And in moving vehicles, I can't look down to read a roadmap, book, or smartphone without nausea quickly following.

When I agreed to be Jordan's rebounding student and test case, I conveniently forgot that my inner ear—or whatever it is that makes vertigo happen—might have some substantial issues with what I'd be asking my body to do.

But having committed to doing this, I follow instructions and begin by gently rocking back and forth on my feet, from my toes to my heels. After just a short while, I notice that my feet are starting to rise up and then sink down into the mat.

Just a wee bit more with every rocking motion, and soon my feet are bouncing up and down slightly off the rebounder mat, almost of their own volition.

Before I realize it, my arms start moving up and down in tandem with my slowly rising and falling feet.

A Spot-On Solution for Dealing with Dizzy

This is actually quite fun, except for one little thing: I'm indeed starting to feel a bit dizzy.

I stop myself from moving and cautiously step off the rebounder and back onto the wooden floor. The dizziness passes quickly, so I step back onto my rebounder to try and get acclimated. The next five minutes are easier. And the following five minutes are even better yet.

Then I realize why!

I've unconsciously started to "spot." That is, I've chosen a spot on the wall directly opposite me to keep looking at while I bounce up and down.

Of course! I'm a dancer, after all, and in my long-ago ballet classes I learned how to spot while doing spins and pirouettes to keep my body stable, graceful, and secure.

It worked then, and sure enough, it's working now.

It makes perfect sense to me that when one is bouncing, the secret to ease, stability, and conquering vertigo is keeping your focus right in front of you. And, most important, *do not look down,* since that's exactly what triggers vertigo, dizziness, and other uncomfortable feelings.[3]

I quickly learn to simply trust that my feet, legs, and body all know what they're doing as I'm bouncing. Little kids learn to bounce easily without overthinking it, and I can too!

WHAT I LEARNED THIS WEEK:

- Trust in yourself, and trust in the act of bouncing on a rebounder.
- Don't be afraid to make use of other things you've learned in the past—like "spotting," warming up, and stretching.
- Choose a spot in the path of your direct forward or upward gaze. Concentrate your attention there. Don't look down at your feet to check if you're balanced. Allow yourself to *feel* the balance instead.
- Begin slowly—no more than five minutes at a time. Then repeat those few minutes as often as you like.
- And always get on and off the mat slowly, carefully, and consciously. If the phone or doorbell rings, do not leap off to get it!

Week 2:
Moving and Meditating Throughout My Day

‖ *Upping My Time, Sinking Down into the Mat*

Following Jordan's instructions, I gradually increase my bouncing time by small increments each day.

---

3   Some sage advice: Never say to yourself—in your head, aloud, or especially aloud to others—"I think if I look down I might fall off..." and then ***actually*** look down. Doing this can distract you and break your stride, and easily make you fall off.

I put myself on a schedule of three bounce sessions a day, which slowly but surely builds up muscle strength in my calves and thighs, and increases my feet's flexibility. I pay close attention to the moment when my fatigued muscles start feeling sore. As soon as I reach the sore point during any given bounce session, I make sure to rest for a bit.

To avoid stepping on and off the mat surface during these short rest sessions, I've learned to incorporate short meditative rests right where I am. I bounce until too much muscle soreness builds up, and then I slow myself down and carefully sink down on the rebounder mat into my favorite cross-legged meditation pose. It's quite comfy to sit on, and certainly feels far better than meditating on a hard floor.

Literally meditating on how my body and mind are feeling in between each bit of bouncing has proven very instructive and useful. For example, I've become aware of what it feels like—the actual sensation—when my muscles relax. After a brief meditative rest stop, I can tell when they're sufficiently rested and ready to go again.

Throughout this week I've fallen into a pattern of five minutes bouncing, two or three minutes meditating, then 10 minutes bouncing. Then another little break, sinking down onto the mat to rest and meditate, then another 10 minutes of bouncing. It all feels perfectly natural and easy.

A Magical Moment, an Already Stronger Me

After one of my meditation breaks I experience a distinctly magical moment. I am dealing with an emotionally difficult day and evening. Without getting into personal details, suffice it to say I'm feeling like a big bag of emotional shite.

I bounce for a while, grateful just to be off on my own, alone in my rebounding space.

A rebounder is designed for and only works well with one person. (Bouncing with two or more people is generally unsafe and not recommended.) So when I'm bouncing, it's just me. It's a perfect place to retreat from whatever else might be concerning me, at least for a little while, and escape the stress and trouble of my day. My rebounder has become a sanctuary, my "safe place."

A mere seven days into being a test case and I can feel how much stronger I am and how my aerobic capacity has dramatically improved. I like how I'm feeling, and I also like that I'm no longer the least bit dizzy or unstable. Also, my tolerance for reading maps in moving cars has apparently increased substantially—I've got my motion sickness on the run! An unexpected and wonderful side effect!

WHAT I LEARNED THIS WEEK:

- Become "body aware" to avoid any possibility of injury from over-indulging in the pure thrill of bouncing, especially when you're just learning.
- Understand that body, mind, emotions, and spirit are all deeply interconnected.
- The simple act of bouncing up and down—being literally airborne nearly half the time—can have the effect of bringing all those pieces of who we are together.
- Children love to bounce on their beds. When we are excited we jump up and down, but have to stop pretty soon because the ground is hard. Bouncing is simply a happy thing to do. And when you do it, you *feel* happy. Obvious, but still remarkable!

Week 3:
Getting in the Groove,
Physically and with Music

‖ Feeling Good Every Day!

I begin most days with a quick five or 10 minutes of the Bounce in the morning, before I leave for work. With my circulation pumping, my mind nicely awake, and my mood rather bright and cheery, I'm totally ready to take on the day.

As willing as I was to become a rebound exercise test case, I had absolutely no idea that I would enjoy it so much! Remember that since childhood and forever after I have never liked to or looked forward to anything called "exercise."

So now we come full circle to my absolute delight in discovering that I actually *like* to exercise! It feels great to bounce up and down, do jumping jacks, run in place, twist, use light hand weights, and much more.

Me, of all people, looking forward to and positively enjoying exercise! Who would have thunk it?

‖ Scheduling My Bounces and Other Logistics

I schedule my rebounding sessions around meals. It's not a good idea to rebound on a freshly full tummy. It doesn't feel very good physically—and you can just imagine what *might* come up (yuck).

I make sure to get some bouncing time in as soon as I return home from work each afternoon. And during the evening, I take little five- or 10-minute bouncing breaks. It's so easy to fit into my already busy life. I put on some favorite music and bounce through three or four songs. Or I watch TV while bouncing. I'm surprised how quickly and easily music or TV makes time flow by.

I was concerned at first that the ceilings in my house might be too low, that I might bounce too high and hit my head. Nope, the ceiling height is not a problem.

A little bit of the Bounce here, a little bit of the Bounce there.

In good weather I can pick up the rebounder and move it out onto the deck. Then I can bounce outdoors in the fresh air, with the sun and the breezes, and under the moon. Plus no ceiling at all but sky. Cool!

My times at the Bounce are getting much longer.

I play my favorite songs in the background as I rebound. Music adds a *lot* of fun and energy. And it gives me an easy way to judge how long I've been bouncing. I find when I promise myself to make it all the way through to the end of a song, I can always push onward just that little bit longer.

WHAT I LEARNED THIS WEEK:
- Even if you've never before been interested in exercise—or you've failed to stick with an exercise program or commitment—rebounding may be a perfect fit for you. For me, rebounding is so easy and so much fun that exercise no longer feels like a burden; it has instead become something I actually look forward to!
- Music makes everything in life so much better, and with rebounding it sets the pace, enhances coordination, and helps me keep track of time.
- Consider bouncing outdoors now and again if you can.

Week 4:
Bouncing Longer with Many Movements and Even Hand Weights!

A Weighty Decision

Now I'm up to fifteen to twenty minutes at a time without getting tired. My endurance, however, depends in part on my choosing music that is really good to listen to as well as functionally appropriate for bouncing. I'm picking longer and longer songs. If it's just two verses away from the finish, I know that all I need to do is hang in there. I now usually make it right through all the songs I've picked.

Jordan suggests that using hand weights—very light ones at first—will add a whole new dimension to bouncing. It will likely make me stronger and probably more muscular. He also says that when you're holding on to light hand weights, there are many different and interesting movements and ways to bounce that naturally suggest themselves.

So this past weekend I went ahead and bought some light hand weights: a two-pound pair and a four-pound pair.

Who Wants More Muscle? ("I do! I do!")

I'm pretty excited about actively building some muscle in my arms. Some of my friends, including men and women my age with gym memberships, have gotten all buff and toned-looking. I know it's possible for me too, and it's likely I have some pretty good genes. But once again, working out on machines at a gym looks to me like way too much work: all sweat, not a lot of fun, and just not worth it.

I realize, obviously, that other folks see it differently and welcome hard workouts at a gym. But that's not for me! I'm a Lazy Girl who'd rather relax and read a good book!

Pretty soon, every time I bounce I'm using the two-pound weights for about half of each song. I'm astonished how light they feel!

The airborne simulated anti-gravity effect of bouncing up and down on the rebounder makes it easy to almost automatically raise and lower the weights. I don't have to think about it, and I'm not consciously expending much more energy than when I'm not using weights. It may seem odd to say this, but it feels like my body came preprogrammed to know how to do this with weights.

I also use hand weights to help focus my attention on such things as the positioning of my arms, feet, and pelvis, and my overall posture and align-ment. (Jordan regularly reminds me of the importance of being aware of the entirety of my body's big picture whenever I'm bouncing.) I very much like this new way of bouncing with weights!

❙ My Basic Movements

This seems like a good time for me to spell out exactly what kinds of movements I typically do when bouncing.

In the beginning days—still less than a month ago!—much of the time I simply gently bounced up and down, not going very high at all and often not leaving the mat entirely. But soon my arms would follow the pattern of my legs, as they opened and closed, up and down, resulting in a classic "jumping jack." It was fun, natural, and easy, and I didn't really even have to think about it.

Then I began running in place on the rebounder. Interestingly, I feel like I'm actually moving forward and not just staying in one place. I love that unlike running on the hard ground, I can run like this without jarring or stressing my knees or ankles. (A good rebounder, I'm told, absorbs up to 80% of the shock that your knees and ankles would otherwise be subject to.)

And then there's bouncing from left to right, doing twists, and rotating my whole body partly or all the way around on the mat. All of these movements make nice horizontal or side-to-side additions on top of my up-and-down movements. Making big arm circles while bouncing feels really wonderful. It releases so much of the tension that I habitually hold in my shoulders and neck.

I also really enjoy a kind of slapping motion—open-hand slapping of my thighs, stomach, and even butt in time to inspiring musical moments. As I become a human percussion instrument, I make some great noises! So much fun! And I really don't care what anybody else hears or thinks!

Last but not least, I often enjoy a simple mellow, up-and-down bounce with my arms held open to the sky, invoking health and good blessings for everyone I know.

WHAT I LEARNED THIS WEEK:
- Use the magic of music while bouncing to increase your pleasure and—perhaps more important—your stamina and longevity. Specific songs that you like will give you a sense of timing to work with and help you achieve your goals.
- Use light hand weights carefully and mindfully to tone and build upper body muscles and put more of a working "load" on your entire body.
- Be creative with the body movements used while bouncing. Experiment, do what moves you, and let yourself be guided by how your body feels in real time.

Week 5:
Everybody Needs a Vacation

Absence Makes the Heart Grow Fonder

This week we are away on summer holidays, traveling through British Columbia. Lots of family get-together dinners, and a big wedding (with a massive feast!) as well.

But alas, there's no rebounder for me to bounce on: I couldn't bring it on the plane and had to leave it at home in Calgary. And dang it, I really I miss it! If we had been driving instead of flying, I'd have duct-taped it to the roof of my car, if need be, just to not be without it. How could I *not* miss it, when happy bouncing has become such a reliable and enjoyable part of my everyday routine?

Well, miss it I did—and more that I would have ever guessed. Sure, I went on many a lovely beach walk on Vancouver Island with my sister-in-law. Yes, I did stretches and moved my body each day. But it just wasn't the same, and compared with my now customary daily rebounding practice, not nearly enough.

Also, alas, I basically gained a pound per day by overeating all that amazing holiday event food. That is, 10 days gone, and 10 pounds gained.

I'm curious to discover how long it will take for those pounds to melt away when I return home and resume my regular practice of the Bounce.

WHAT I LEARNED THIS WEEK:
- Don't despair if your usual exercise schedule is interrupted by circumstance. Just do whatever you can, and look forward to picking up from wherever you left off. And eat all that great holiday food guilt free! That's what a good vacation is for. You can likely bounce it all off as soon as you return home!

Week 6: Back in Gear

‖ Making Up for Missed Time

After arriving home on Sunday night, I dropped my suitcase in the front hallway and went straight to my rebounder. I expected my muscle tone and stamina to have decreased somewhat during my 10 days away, and indeed that was the case. It was most noticeable on that first night, but by the following day, and certainly the day after that, I was mostly back up to speed.

While my legs did miss being properly worked out, I'd already built up some good strong leg muscles, and was surprised and pleased at how rapidly they recovered.

‖ Breathing Better Increases Stamina and Pleasure

This week, I'm working on building aerobic stamina by being much more conscious of my breathing patterns while bouncing. Like many people—both on and off the rebounder—I have a tendency to hold my breath for extended periods of time. With the kind of focus I've been putting into my bouncing movements and routines, I wasn't very surprised to notice I'd been intermittently holding my breath.

To counter this tendency, I've been practicing visualizing my breathing mechanism as a vital piece of the rebounding puzzle. When I'm breathing consciously, my mind focuses much better on what the rest of my body is doing.

I've started making a few videos of myself bouncing happily to some of my favorite songs. It's interesting to watch myself. When I describe myself as "bouncing happily" I'm being quite literal.

I can feel a smile growing on my face. With each cycle of rising and falling and rising up again, my grin widens. Watching myself on video—from the outside looking in—is mesmerizing, instructive, and lots of fun.

Being the dedicated teacher he is, Jordan created and sent me some new bouncing videos by email. A quick mouse click and there he is on my screen, instructing me and being very encouraging. It's great fun for me to play and replay his examples until I feel like I'm mirroring each move in real time. Video lessons are so useful!

Whenever I'm bouncing, I'm also smiling—big time. This happens not just because I'm feeling happy or because the very act of bouncing up and down is so much fun. In fact, I experience a kind of super-smile that feels like it comes from deep inside of me and then pops out of its own volition. I almost feel like I'm outside myself, watching the smile blossom and grow, making me healthier, happier, and stronger.

By the end of this week I'm often continuously bouncing for twenty minutes or more each session. I work up quite a sweat and drink a whole lot of water before and after bouncing. But hey! Not only *can* I do this, I *am* doing this! Woot! And it's great.

WHAT I LEARNED THIS WEEK:
- Once a certain fitness level is attained through rebounding, it is gratifying to see that it can be quickly recovered following a period of inactivity.
- Once you become aware that your aerobic capacity has begun to increase, keep in mind that it can substantially improve even more as time passes, especially if you consistently place attention on your breath.
- Bouncing seems to never get boring or become less fun. There's so much variety in what you can do with such a seemingly simple exercise instrument.
- It's very important to breathe well and remain conscious of your breathing while bouncing. Once you set your body in a pattern of breathing at the start of a session, you can then pretty much forget about it. Your body takes over from there and happily continues with the pattern you've set in place, leaving you free to focus on other things.

Week 7:
Getting Fitter and Stronger

Quadrupling My Time!

Since the holidays, I've been back in the comfort zone of my daily bounce practice for a full week.

My aerobic capacity is right back up to where it was before my holiday break. Indeed, this week I've been actively testing my stamina to see just how long I can continuously bounce for without having to stop to rest. Right now, twenty minutes is my comfortable limit. But I can really feel that I'm close to one of those aerobic turning points.

During my first week, a mere five minutes of bouncing totally wore me out. Then, all of a sudden, it didn't wear me out at all! Wheee!!!

Getting stronger and fitter all the time feels really good, and I love being able to track my progress. The clock, my breathing, my energy level—they don't lie. And my lovely new leg muscles, they don't lie either. It's really quite encouraging.

Music Makes It Marvelously Easy

For me at least, the real key to long continuous bouncing sessions is choosing the right music and songs to bounce to.

Bouncing to fast and exciting songs is fabulous. But not surprisingly, going nonstop full tilt wears me out much faster. My solution is to alternate highly stimulating song choices with more mellow music. Even quieter songs with a good beat are nice to bounce to. Indeed, for those not yet ready to push themselves very hard, slower songs are perfect: you still benefit from the aerobic workout, just at a slower and gentler pace.

Also, bouncing to quieter songs is a great opportunity to focus on other important things like balance, stability, and placement of arms and legs in relation to my core body movement. I don't even need to lift off of the mat, just flex my feet gently.

When I have a session with a variety of very energetic songs mixed with slower ones, I find that my stamina increases dramatically. The slower songs offer a bit of a rest period, without completely interrupting my bouncing time. A full half hour now flies by easily.

Finding the Time; Staying Safe

As much as I now love the Bounce, making sure I get in my minimum half an hour on the rebounder each and every day can be really difficult. Life, as we all know, gets in the way and sometimes becomes incredibly busy. Friends and family drop by unexpectedly, and supposedly quiet evenings become social ones. Still, I haven't missed a single day yet—other than when on the road.

Something that should go without saying: do *not* bounce if you've been drinking alcohol or are otherwise unable to bring focus and concentration to a bounce session. And definitely do not let your friends who have been drinking idly "try out" your rebounder during a social evening. I had a friend hop up on my rebounder when he was drunker than he or I realized. He nearly wobbled and bobbled right through the glass panes of the French door next to my rebounder. Safety first! And always!

Nice Developments

I notice that my legs are showing visibly defined muscles now. I can actually see the shape of my calves, and any wobble that might have been in my thighs is no longer there. The same goes for my arms—I have more muscle than ever before. Jordan's system of bouncing with light hand weights is apparently very effective!

It would appear that it really does not take all that long for regular exercise—at least on a rebounder—to provide some appealing changes. I'm thinking that one of the big factors is the "regular" part!

Starting slowly, building up, keeping at it while finding a way to make rebound exercise a daily life habit. I eat. I sleep. I work. I read. I chat online. I practice the Bounce.

WHAT I LEARNED THIS WEEK:
- Keeping track of your progress is very motivating.
- The benefits that accrue from the Bounce are measurable and worth noticing.
- Choose a good variety of fast and slow songs to bounce to.
- Educate your friends that a rebounder is not a toy. It looks like a miniature trampoline, but it's much more than that, and quite different. It is an exercise instrument, and deserves respect. And obviously, rebounding while using booze (or anything that could affect your balance and concentration) is a big no-no.

Week 8: My Times Are Longer, and My Body's Stronger!

Taking Advantage of Muscle Memory

When you bounce over and over again to music that you especially love, the music seeps deep down into your muscle memory. Each time you bounce to a particular song that you know well, your body can then go into a kind of relaxed autopilot mode.

If this is one of those times when your mind needs some pure relaxation, you can just let your muscle memory take over. This frees your creative mind to add in more and different improvised movements and patterns each session. It also gives you the kind of mental spaciousness to let you easily observe your breath, posture, and what the big picture looks while you're bouncing up and down.

This week I'm rebounding happily to a daily schedule of one long session—a full half hour after work each afternoon—and several little five-to-ten-minute bouncing sessions randomly throughout the evening.

Grateful Bouncing Indoors and Out

The weather's very warm here. I'm grateful that I can pick up my rebounder and easily take it out onto my backyard deck, and bounce in the cool of the evening breeze. It weighs about thirty pounds, but now feels a lot lighter than when I first got it, no doubt because I really am significantly stronger now.

I've started asking friends and family to make videos of my bounce sessions. What astonishes me is how much interest people have whenever I post anything rebounding-related on Facebook, especially my little rebounding videos to music. Others seem to be fascinated simply by observing how much pure fun bouncing to great music can be. And there's nothing like watching and listening to a video to prove it!

More and more I deeply believe that Jordan's vision—bringing the magic and pure fun of regular rebound exercise back to public awareness—is not only possible, but inevitable. Folks just need to be exposed to the concept, encouraged to get a decent rebounder, and guided to try it for themselves.

WHAT I LEARNED THIS WEEK:

- As you keep to a comfortable schedule, bouncing becomes so very easy to like. At least in my own case, I can easily reach a point where "Have To" becomes "Want To"—which then transforms into "Want To Very Much!"

- Choosing your favorite songs, and bouncing to them repeatedly, is wonderfully effective. Exercise that's repeated to music you like and know well builds a kind of muscle memory that's both very useful and fascinating to experience. Regularly listening to songs you love can help you set and achieve exercise goals.
- Be brave if a challenge is offered to you! Be willing to go for it. Understand that if you falter, that's still better than not trying at all. Without blame or guilt, you can simply step right back up and get back to the Bounce as soon as you're ready. Success is bound to be in your future if you stay open, do the work, and keep going.

Chapter 3:

Major Physical Benefits of the Bounce

Personal experience and reports from many of our friends (old and new) point to the same thing: the Bounce is a fantastic physical and spiritual practice for nearly anyone who wants to live a long, strong, happy, healthy life.

As already noted, in addition to being highly physically effective, bouncing is also easy, safe, convenient, and inherently fun and enjoyable. Even if you have another primary form of exercise—yoga, dance, walking, tennis, team sports, Pilates, a martial art, swimming, weight training, and so on—non-skeleton-jarring rebounding can be a tremendously beneficial adjunct. The bottom line: the Bounce readily offers a wide range of physical benefits that make it ideal as a primary or supplemental exercise modality.

One Body per Lifetime

We only get one body per lifetime. Sure, modern medical science can do some wonderful things, but none of the fixes it offers will work very well for very long if the body's underlying main structures and systems aren't healthy, strong, and flexible enough to accept, integrate, and work with what's offered.

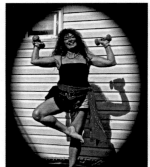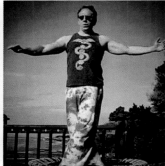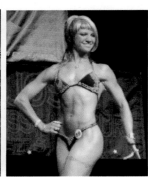

Joy Daniels, Jordan Gruber, and Krisztina Lazar

Like it or not, then, the task of achieving health, longevity, and vigor is still 100% up to each of us individually. Take a moment to reflect, and ask yourself if you're content with how you're treating your body (and how it's treating you).

We all know that exercise is good for us. There always seems to be a new study out or a social media post that confirms this obvious truth. As for rebounding, many claims as to its benefits have been made through the years, some with hard facts behind them, but many others based mostly on wild yet hopeful speculation. Instead of simply recycling those old claims, we're going to present current, fact-based research on health and exercise as well as firsthand personal accounts of how rebounding works and has improved people's lives.

Very importantly, *much of the research we'll present on why exercising benefits everything from mood to weight loss isn't necessarily specific to rebound exercise.* But the research overwhelmingly shows that exercise that provides a combination of cardio activity, strength training, and balance training benefits just about everyone. Well, that's just what bouncing does best: combine these three training modalities in a unique fun way that few other exercise can match. (Another thing bouncing does really well is boost your immune system, which we'll turn to shortly.)

There is also rebounding-specific research that has been done over the years—including an early NASA study and a few recent studies—with strong positive results. On a personal level, your two authors have found rebounding to be highly effective. But instead of just taking our word for it, we want you to consider the research we'll present, the stories we'll tell (our own stories, as well as the stories of friends and correspondents), and the ideas we'll put forth—and then you can decide for yourself.

When you work out regularly, your brain gets used to frequent surges of activity and adapts by turning certain genes on or off. (Note that leaps and bounds, as it were, are regularly being made in what is called "epigenetics," or the study of how particular genes are activated or deactivated by environmental factors and lifestyle choices.) Many of these changes boost brain cell function and protect against diseases such as Alzheimer's, and Parkinson's, and even help ward off injuries and age-related decline.

Science is discovering more and more that exercise is crucial in treating and allowing people to live with chronic conditions and disease. The old way of thinking—that bed rest is the best way to heal most things—no longer holds. In fact, the more sedentary you become, especially when your health is compromised, the more your condition is likely to become worse...sometimes much worse. This doesn't mean, of course, that you should expect to run a marathon when you have terrible leg pain. What studies do show, however, is that what is most beneficial is combining movement, moderate to intense cardio, and strength training. In our experience, rebounding is terrific at doing just that.

Enhanced Lymph Flow and Immune System Function

The best and most effective way to avoid chronic diseases is to have a robust and fully functioning immune system. Bouncing helps move your lymph fluid and thereby keeps your lymphatic system—and therefore your immune system—healthy and strong.

Lymph is a clear or slightly whitish alkaline fluid that originates as interstitial fluid in your body. "Interstitial" means the space between, and in this case the space we're talking about is the space between all the organs, vessels, and tissues inside your body.

Our bodies contain about twice as much lymph as blood, with lymph playing a crucial role in warding off disease and keeping us healthy. The lymph bathes nearly all of our tissues to accomplish three crucial tasks:

- Keeping cells well lubricated
- Keeping cells nourished with nutrients and oxygen, which reach most cells by floating through the lymph fluid
- Keeping cells cleansed and detoxified by clearing away cellular waste, harmful bacteria, and environmental pollution

Lymph gets channeled through the lymphatic system, a bodily system that parallels the circulatory system. Using capillaries that eventually end up at lymph nodes, the lymph system is designed as a filtration system. The lymph comes from your blood vessels, is moved along until it hits a node, gets cleansed and filtered by the white blood cells within the node, and then seeps back into the blood vessels, refreshed and ready to keep going.

The lymphatic system has channels and nodes all over the body. In addition to the nodes and capillaries, specific body organs are principally lymph organs. Thus your bone marrow produces B lymphocytes, a type of immune system cell that makes antibodies (markers for what the immune system needs to destroy) against antigens (external substances that, when they get inside you, are toxic to your cells). Your spleen acts like a large lymph node and serves as a blood filter. Your tonsils and thymus gland produce T lymphocytes (T cells), which play an essential role in fighting disease throughout the body through cell-mediated immunity. There is also a large concentration of lymph tissue surrounding the intestines; this absorbs fats and separates nutrients from pathogens.

However, the lymph system *doesn't constantly and automatically pump* like the circulatory system does! By contrast, the heart continuously pumps blood to keep it moving through the body by applying the pressure necessary to keep things flowing. Your *lymph, on the other hand, only gets moved by muscle contractions*, like from your lungs when you breathe, or from your skeletal muscles when you move. Only whole-body motion keeps the lymph moving throughout your whole body. That's where exercise—bouncing in particular—comes in.

The lymph system is designed to move lymph through the body's own movement. The more you move, the more efficient and effective your lymph system becomes. Stagnation in the lymph causes buildup of cell waste and toxins, which in turn leads to an inhibited immune system and illness. Whether or not it makes visible symptoms outside your body, this clutter of toxins puts your cells into an unhealthy immediate environment, where the pollution and debris block the cells' access to the oxygen, nutrients, and messenger chemicals they need for their ongoing survival.

Lymph moves one-directionally in the body—namely, up from the legs to the base of the neck (recent research shows that there is even a lymph channel that goes into the brain!). That's why up-and-down movement is essential for pumping your lymph. Some types of exercise, such as running, can provide a slight up-and-down movement, and swimming is always great, but there's nothing quite like the built-in gravitational force flux of bouncing to maximize this pumping.[4] Rebounding alternates between providing an experience akin to weightlessness and then an experience of more than the regular 1 g of force we normally feel at the Earth's surface. This contrast of forces in motion—changing many times each minute as you bounce—produces an effective pumping action that enables the lymph system to do its job of bathing the cells and tissues, lubricating them, bringing them nutrients, and removing and disposing waste products.

The lymph system and immune system are very closely interrelated. The immune system works in part by utilizing the lymph system to protect your body against disease and damaging foreign bodies. When functioning properly, the immune system identifies viruses, bacteria, parasites, fungi, cancerous tumors, and a variety of other threats. The immune system identifies these threats and works to distinguish unwelcome intruders within your body so they can be addressed.

---

4   Bonnie Annis, in her article "Rebounding for Lymphedema," writes: "The lymph fluid moves through channels called 'vessels' that are filled with one-way valves, so it always moves in the same direction. The main lymph vessels run up the legs, up the arms and up the torso. This is why the vertical up-and down movement of rebounding is so effective to pump the lymph." It is often asserted that it the pressure differential experienced at the top of the bounce mechanically accounts for how rebounding actually pumps lymph fluid through this series of one-way valves.

Recognize your immune system as your body's protective army. The overall mobility of that army is based on your immune system's ability to travel through the lymph system and regroup as needed to defend your body against invaders. If your army is weighed down by limited mobility and poor communication, it won't be able to mobilize quickly and effectively. But if it is supple, light, and agile, and has good communication, its troops can identify, mobilize, and deal with any enemy much more efficiently.

The movement at the heart of any regular bounce practice keeps your lymph system functioning properly. Rebounding daily keeps your agile protector troops always on the move, training new recruits, and bringing the forces of healing promptly to where they are most needed. In a world of viral pandemics, having as strong and vital an immune system as you can readily manage makes a lot of sense, and rebounding is among the very best and easiest means of accomplishing this.

Better Balance

> Think of balance in general: The ground is very flat, and we live on very predictable surfaces. We stuff our feet into shoes, and therefore our feet are not really connected to our vestibular system and our balance. If your feet are not being challenged, you're pruning away your body's natural ability to balance well.
>
> That's why a good rebounder is such a great thing: You can do simple bouncing on it with one foot, switch legs, and much more, and all those things help develop your balance in a really nice way. It also strengthens your pelvis and your hips.
>
> —Tom McCook, Director, Center of Balance, Mountain View, California

Our constantly in-motion bodies rebalance themselves in relation to our environment and the other parts of our bodies. Even when we seem to be sitting or standing still, micro-movements that we use to readjust ourselves are happening continuously.

Balance enhancement is another foundational element of exercise readily provided by rebound exercise. Both stationary balance (the ability to be in a still poised position—for example, standing on both legs) and dynamic balance (the ability to move and change directions on varying surfaces under different conditions) are very important to how we live our lives, especially as we grow older and balance becomes more of an issue. Rebounding helps with both of these balance modalities, so we'll discuss them together.

As we grow older, distinct changes to our balance ability become more evident. The ability to keep our balance and stay sure-footed becomes an increasing challenge that many people don't see coming. And when it does come, many find it quite unnerving. As a teenager, perhaps you could successfully walk on a balance beam, but now something as simple as quickly turning on your feet can be a problem. Moreover, balance issues are the single greatest reason for falls and injuries in the elderly.

Now, many people believe that the deterioration of balance—to the point of dysfunction and injury—is one of those things that *has* to happen to you when you get older. It happened to your grandparents and parents, so it must also happen to you, right? Nope. Not so. Balance is something you can work on and improve no matter how old you are. The belief that falls should be accepted and tolerated as part of the aging process is a myth that needs dispelling. Many if not most falls can and should be prevented.

Balance comes from your muscles' ability to keep you steady. This means that there must necessarily be a collaborative effort that cascades through your muscular, skeletal, and nervous systems each time you take a step— or, when you get right down to it, make any movement at all. Through regular physical training, this collaboration becomes better synced and harmonized, not to mention stronger. How exactly do you strengthen it? When you push yourself to the limit—safely—all of your collaborating systems naturally work together harder, better, and more efficiently.

> I'm 72 and have had a balance problem since experiencing an inner ear issue in 2011. Because of asthma and mild chronic obstructive pulmonary disease, I could only walk

in the spring and fall due to higher heat and biting cold. I decided to purchase a bungee-based rebounder with a support bar, knowing I could return them if they didn't work out.

It was the best gift I have given myself to date! The results in only two months have been more energy and stamina, and an improvement in balance and coordination. My chiropractor said it was the best purchase that I could have made for myself because it positively affects every cell in my body.

My massage therapist said that she could tell the difference in my legs and butt already; I'm hoping that it happens to my upper body also. I feel so much more confident with my inner ear balance issues and want to let my physical therapist know that I recommend rebounding for anyone with a balance issue. Thank you for all your help, and I'm just sorry that I didn't start sooner.

—Faye Lewark Daniels

Let's consider an example. When you first stand on a rebounder, you may notice that your feet need to constantly adjust themselves to keep your body erect. These many muscles movements are training your brain and body in real time to balance better and to adjust to the new environment your body is experiencing. Acting and feeling like the single connected organism that it actually is, your body is rewiring your neural pathways to become more efficient as your sensory-motor control becomes smoother and more cohesive. (This is the same process for building any new skill pathway, such as practicing touching the end of your nose with your fingertip.)

During this process, your mind and body come to work better as a whole unit, and your brain improves its ability to keep track of where your limbs are at all times, which translates into fewer stumbles, less clumsiness, and ultimately fewer falls.

Body imbalances can also cause bodily tension and be related to balance degeneration. From an embryological standpoint, your feet can be considered part of your lower back.[5] When one or more links in the chain of movement are missing or impaired, the entire chain is compromised, and soreness and pain usually result somewhere.

Balance-strengthening exercise also helps prevent injuries to the anterior cruciate ligament (ACL) in the human knee, and has been proven to reduce the rate of ankle sprains. Better balance helps strengthen muscles, ligaments, and tendons, as well as increasing general body awareness. Improving and strengthening balance is an extremely effective way not only to rehabilitate injuries, but to prevent them in the first place.

Unlike steady ground or most of the floors we walk on every day, a rebounder creates an environment of controlled instability—ever changing but perfectly manageable. This exposes your body and mind to a series of multisensory challenges. By developing ever-improvised new responses, you improve your balance and neuromuscular control. All of this is a fancy way of saying that when you proactively create safe but challenging balance conditions that your body must adjust to, your brain sends signals to your muscles to adapt to the new conditions and creates new pathways. This in turn makes your entire integrated body/mind smarter. And who wouldn't want that?

Building Strength, Muscle Tone, and Muscle

The fascinating thing about bouncing is that it seems to help your own unique body reach its individualized perfect form. If you need to lose

---

5   As embodiment teacher Tom McCook has pointed out, our feet are meant for different surfaces—mud, sand, rocks, forest floor, grasslands, etc. They are designed to adjust, balance, and adapt to the variation found in these different landscapes, just as our overall musculature and bodies are designed to adapt and compensate through nearly constant adjustments. Unfortunately, most of us wear shoes nearly all the time, and very rarely do our shoes challenge our feet in any significant way. Even worse, too much of the time our shoes are not just limiting, but downright uncomfortable (either for fashion's sake or because we take our feet for granted and don't bother to make sure they're comfortable). But when our feet are stuffed into shoes that restrict adaptation and movement, those shoes become deprivation (if not torture) chambers. Essentially, by wearing most types of shoes, and by wearing them for so much of our awake time, we make our bodies less intelligent by rarely challenging our feet, and in turn our balance grows weaker.

weight—you will. It you need to gain weight—you will. Of course, it's not your weight on the scale but how toned and strong you become (and how well your clothes fit) that really counts. As we have had to point out to many people—even Joy needed to work this one through in her head at first—muscle weighs more than fat, so if you become much fitter by losing fat and gaining muscle, your weight could stay the same...or even increase!

Strength is another foundational structural element provided by rebound exercise. Formally defined, strength is the ability of the neuromuscular system to produce internal tension in the muscles and connective tissue that pull on bone, and thereby to overcome an external force. Traditionally, strength training has focused on developing the greatest amount of strength in a single plane of motion, like in most bodybuilding exercises.

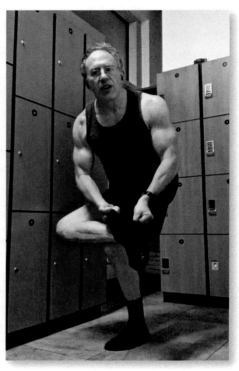

Jordan at 60!

However, focusing only on developing muscles without increasing the whole-body fitness of one's joints and connective tissues—as well as blood and lymph circulation and oxygen distribution throughout the body—tends to result in inconsistently developed muscles with limited ability of the whole body to support and use those stronger muscles. That is, the muscles may be stronger in isolated exercise, but the body has not become stronger overall. Such imbalanced development can in turn lead to injuries. Obviously, this is not a healthy or wise approach to overall fitness for a lifetime.

Importantly, as the National Academy of Sports Medicine teaches, strength can't be thought of in isolation, but must be built on a foundation of stabilization. As a building's foundation balances multiple forces, for example with the use of both concrete and steel in a skyscraper, a healthy fitness foundation requires the collaboration of muscles, tendons, and ligaments throughout the body.

Building strength through rebounding or any other means, then, isn't primarily about increasing muscle tone or size (although rebounding can do a great job at this, as we've experienced ourselves and will discuss later). Instead, the importance of building and maintaining strength is mainly about *making you strong for your daily life*. You need strength to move things (and simply to move), to take out the garbage, to vacuum, to do any number of activities that can become difficult or ultimately impossible if your body loses substantial muscle and muscle tone. Thus, increased whole-body strength and balance both makes difficult tasks feasible and ordinary everyday life easier to flow through with plenty of ongoing energy.

A holistic approach to building strength is needed to support a commitment to your body's long-term health. Such balanced development is an absolutely essential component of physical activity as we age. When you bounce on a rebounder, you will not only get a great cardiorespiratory workout, but can also easily, effectively, and safely build your strength. For example, you can build significant strength just by moving your own body weight, and we suggest a variety of ways to do this in later chapters on specific types of rebound exercise movements and workouts.

With the constant pull of rhythmically pulsed—increased and decreased—gravity from the up-and-down motion of your body on a rebounder, you're making your muscles work both differently and arguably more than they would in a standard terrestrial workout. Couple that with an increase in heart rate and fuller joint rotation, and you're very quickly taking your activity to a whole new level.

Suppose you're interested in toning your muscles, or building muscle to become more "buff" generally? Can you get substantially bigger, buffer, and stronger with rebounding? Let's look at the biophysics. To begin with, every time you bounce you're activating and challenging the musculature (including the associated ligaments and tendons) in your legs and core, and every time you move one of your arms about, you're moving around an "object" that weighs between five and fifteen pounds. Furthermore, by using hand weights—which, held at arm's length, are leveraged through your shoulder to provide a lot of work—and other resistive devices, you can also treat yourself to an invigorating and rigorous upper-body bouncing workout.

But how effective will it be? Let's consider the ideas of James White, Ph.D., in his 1984 book *Jump for Joy: The Rebounding Exercise Book*. Dr. White, former director of research and rehabilitation in the physical education department at the University of California at San Diego (UCSD), explained how "jumping for health" offers the muscles a true physical strengthening effect: "Rebounding allows the muscles to go through the full range of motion at equal force. It helps people learn to shift their weight properly and to be aware of body positions and balance."

An advocate of rebounding for athletic conditioning, White used the rebounder in his UCSD rehabilitation program. "When you jump, jog, and twist on this [jumping] device, you can exercise for hours without getting tired. It's great practice for skiing, it improves your tennis stroke, and it's a good way to burn off calories and lose weight," he writes. White adds that "jumping for health" is more effective for fitness and weight loss than cycling, running, or jogging, and it has the added advantage of producing fewer injuries.

In addition to Dr. White's ideas on why rebounding is so effective, later on (in chapter 8's "Jordan's Journal") we'll discuss a number of different factors that help explain why the Bounce can be so effective at toning and building muscle. These include:

- The "physics of fitness" and how understanding your body as a system of levers and pulleys helps explains both how challenging rebounding can be and how to take advantage of the opportunities it affords;
- The eccentric—and therefore very effective at muscle toning and building—contractions that rebounding makes use of;
- The way you can intelligently and thoroughly reach muscle failure— necessary to build muscle—by using light weights; and
- The benefits of entering the 3D/4D Vitruvian Sphere, as already mentioned.

By combining all of these factors, our experience is that the Bounce is *very* effective at toning and building muscle. With just the slightest twist of your arm or shoulder here, the progressive use of weights to safely increase the load you're bearing there, and a commitment to conscious breathing and to keep moving through more and more of the potential space available to you, your muscles really *can* get a thorough workout that produces some pretty amazing results. Both of your authors, Jordan (starting at age 42) and Joy (starting at age 59), gained over twenty pounds of skeletal muscle in their first three years of bouncing. You can see some of our pictures both in this book and online.

One last thing about muscle toning and strengthening that's of particular interest to women—especially those who have given birth—is that bouncing also often has a positive effect on bladder control and other internal bodily functions. We'll say more about this in chapters 4 and 7.

Aerobic/Cardiovascular Fitness

Cardiorespiratory fitness (CRF) reflects the ability of the circulatory and respiratory systems to supply oxygen-rich blood to skeletal muscles during sustained physical activity. Or, in other words, to get your breathing and heart rate up by moving your body so that your muscles get much-needed blood. Sometimes it's referred to as cardiovascular fitness, referring to the heart and the blood vessels; sometimes it's referred to as cardiorespiratory fitness, referring to the overall circulatory system's distribution of blood, and the lungs bringing oxygen from the air we breathe into the blood while moving carbon dioxide out of the blood to the air as we breathe out.

Call it what you want, it's an absolutely necessity for the body. Along with strength, balance, and a strong immune system, it's a "must have" for being a physically healthy human being. The nearly endless benefits of cardiorespiratory fitness include:

- A stronger and more efficient heart generally, meaning improved ability to pump blood (enhance cardiac output)
- Improved blood thinning and reduced risk of clot formation
- Improved ability of muscles to use oxygen

- Improved tolerance for stress
- Improved sleep and ability to relax
- Increase in lean body mass
- Increase in metabolic rate and ability to burn calories
- Stronger respiratory muscles (like the intercostal muscles between your ribs)
- More efficient breathing and improved lung capacity, therefore a lower heart rate for the same beneficial distribution of oxygen throughout your body
- Reduced risk of heart disease
- Reduced cholesterol
- Reduced arterial blood pressure
- Reduced risk of obesity and diabetes

There are many ways you can get good cardio exercise on a rebounder. You can sprint, run in place, do jumping jacks, dance, bounce in circles, and anything else your imagination comes up with as you spontaneously move your body. The simple act of bouncing easily provides an aerobic workout. When you incorporate moving your arms, you've created a much more efficient whole-body aerobic workout. And if you use light hand weights, you work harder and get more benefits all the way around.

Think of what most people consider a cardio workout: running. What do you do when you run? You move forward in a single direction, moving your legs a lot while minimally swinging your arms for momentum. That's it. The entire rest of your body is minimally engaged in keeping you upright and moving forward, but not much else is going on.

Now picture a rebounder. When you bounce up and down on it and move your arms, your entire body is engaged in multidimensional movement. Your joints move in a variety of directions as you experience your body moving through a much fuller range of motion. Your heart is pumping blood to all of your body, and as you move you're helping your lymph circulate throughout your entire body more efficiently as well.

You're not, then, just engaged in a repetitive, singular forward motion, where you pound your feet into the ground (or the treadmill), jarring your joints over and over again. Instead, you're engaging your entire body in a non-jarring supportive way that lubricates your joints, bathes your organs, and oxygenates your muscles in an efficient manner. We think this all sounds pretty good—and it feels even better.

Weight Maintenance and Management

Bouncing makes a distinct positive difference in losing and managing weight, and in maintaining high personal energy levels. You can make use of rebounding as your primary physical exercise practice, or incorporate it into your current exercise routine, program, or lifestyle.

Many people may pick up this book because they desire to lose some weight—to become a little slimmer, to lose some flab, to look their best. While changing your food intake—the quality and quantity of what you consume—makes a big difference, it at best addresses half the equation, because it doesn't include calories burned through activity. Our bodies are meant to move. Our physical being literally falls apart—or, more typically, ossifies and becomes immobile, painful, and dysfunctional—when we are sedentary, and our risk for disease skyrockets. There's no way around it: to speed up your metabolic rate and burn more calories, you simply have to move more.

Your metabolism—the process that converts what you eat and drink into energy—is directly related to weight loss. While research shows that our metabolism tends to slow down with age, some simple changes can boost your metabolism, including:

- Moving more throughout the day and becoming less sedentary generally;
- Improving your cardiovascular fitness with aerobic exercise; and
- Building skeletal muscle, since muscle tissue burns more calories than does fat.

All of these changes are easy to implement with a rebounder. You can bounce multiple times a day, increasing your movement-to-stillness ratio to boost your metabolism. Since bouncing on a rebounder is also inherently aerobic, you can purposefully increase your heart rate by doing intervals, jogging, sprinting, moving your arms, and moving your whole body.

Moreover, by incorporating handheld weights and other types of resistive bouncing equipment, you can dramatically increase the positive effects of rebound exercise (as well as your heart rate). You'll not only burn more calories as you bounce, but build core strength as well as working a variety of muscle groups. All of this creates and maintains lean, strong muscle to help keep you mobile, strong, and properly aligned as you age.

Keep in mind that exercise needs to be fun—it has to be something you really enjoy—if you're going to spend 30 to 60 minutes a day doing it. And that's one of the beauties of rebounding that really takes things to the next level: it's a safe and sustainable exercise regimen that's endlessly challenging and actually really fun! When you experiment with different kinds of music or watch TV shows (or talk on the phone with headphones or earbuds), the possibilities are virtually endless.

By following our guidelines, you can establish an enjoyable rebounding practice that builds strength, endurance, and fitness without injury. Then, as you expand your physical capabilities—your strength, range of motion, balance, and endurance—you can introduce different kinds of movements and equipment (like a set of progressive handheld weights) to keep yourself engaged, stimulated, and challenged in a variety of ways.

Easy Automatic Cross-Training

We all need regular physical activity to be healthy and productive. Human beings do best—stay healthiest, thrive, and have the most fun—when our regular ongoing schedules incorporate a wide range of real-world activities requiring a wide variety of physical motions and movements.

Building cross-training into our everyday lives makes common sense, and the wide variety of movements, motions, and physical configurations made possible by the Bounce makes rebound exercise a perfect way to supercharge your regular routine for life. That is, if you add in bouncing to your existing routine, you're adding in a robust cross-training element that will benefit you across multiple dimensions.

What does that look like? The variety of movements you can do on a rebounder is almost infinite, and you're in total control of the intensity—how hard and how long you bounce. You can pulse up and down, you can run or dance, or you can bounce so gently that your feet never leave the mat, all the while moving your arms in countless ways, from jumping jacks to arm circles to hand dancing to clapping.[6] And as you will see, you can move using only your body or you can use light hand weights, Shake Weights, plastic resistance bands (such as TheraBands), weighted gloves, and more.

Increasing Baseline Movement to Leverage Long-Term Health

Both cardiovascular fitness and ideal weight maintenance require each of us to have sufficient movement in our lives. That is, on average, we each need to sufficiently move our one and only body every single day. Such movement helps keep us healthy, prevents injury, and sends our physical systems, organs, and genes the right kinds of signals. Therefore, finding a way to maintain or increase our baseline movement statistics—especially as we age—is of critical importance. (Many smartphones and dedicated fitness watches and monitors provide detailed fitness and activity information in terms of daily steps, calories burned, heart rate averages, maximums and minimums, and so on.)

There's no question that each of us needs to incorporate sufficient move-ment and exercise into our daily lives, but for those past a certain age without an existing exercise program, activity, or mindset that seamlessly

---

6   The list of what you can do on or with a rebounder is huge, with virtually endless combinations and possibilities. However, since we're well aware that endless pos-sibilities can be overwhelming, there are specific chapters dedicated to helping you get started with some basic movements and routines as well as advising you on how to continually make progress.

works for them, this may not be so easy.[7] There are, of course, a wide variety of activities, some of which are particularly good at giving whole-body workouts, like gymnastics, certain martial arts, and swimming. So if you have something you like or love and can get it done, terrific! Keep going!

But if you don't already have something like this in your life, please remember that it's never too late to get in shape and become healthier. No matter what you look like or feel like right now, if it's not something that you prefer or that pleases you, you don't have to accept it as something that just inevitably happens to you because you're getting older.

Whether you work full time, are a stay-at-home parent, are in school, or are fully or partially retired, it's not too late to begin your own regular bounce practice and start to feel the benefits so readily and reliably available to you.

Once you've received clearance from your doctor or health expert and have obtained a decent-quality rebounder, please make sure to take the time to go slow and give it your best shot. If you're feeling bad, there's a good chance—as backed by science and the experience of many people—that you may start feeling a whole lot better physically. And if you're feeling a whole lot better about yourself physically, then your mind, heart, and emotions are surely bound to follow along and soon feel better as well.

---

7   Gyms can be intimidating and confusing, and hiring a trainer can be very expensive. Incorrectly using gym equipment (machines and especially free weights) or going at it too hard (e.g., having an overzealous trainer) can cause injury and substantially set you back. Many people default to running or walking outside, but when bad weather hits, exercise commitments quickly fade. Plus, the stress of literally pounding the pavement can be very detrimental to one's bones, joints, and connective tissue. So for many people, especially as they get older, running is simply no longer feasible and sustainable. Yoga and Pilates are wonderful, but often it's hard to get in more than a class or maybe two a week—and that's just not enough. Similarly, some people do their favorite outdoor sport or activity—like biking, hiking, or playing tennis or basketball—at least once or sometimes twice a weekend, but again, that's just not enough.

Chapter 4:

A Guide to Gear, Safety, and Setting Up

What it takes to bounce well is simple: a good rebounder and an appropriate place to use it, a few accessories to maximize your workouts, a safety-first focus, and not much else. This chapter considers first rebounders themselves, and then some essential accessories. It then turns to the all-important subject of safety, before focusing on how to actually—physically—set up and get ready for bouncing.

Gear, safety, and setup are three legs of one larger focus: getting the greatest benefits from bouncing as safely, easily, and effectively as possible. If you develop good habits early on—such as learning to super-quickly check how tight your rebounder's legs are screwed on, making sure you've got water nearby, and having a plan for what to do when your phone demands your attention—things will go more smoothly, you'll enjoy bouncing more, and you'll receive more of the benefits that sustained bouncing provides.

Gear: What You'll Need and What You Might Want

Rebounder: You'll Need a Decent One Even If You've Got a Trampoline

To some extent, you can get a rebounding-like workout—at least as far as the lymphatic and aerobic benefits go—using any of the following kinds of equipment or objects:

- Beds and other objects with springs
- Bounce-back chairs
- Pogo sticks
- Jump Boots (e.g., Kangoo Jumps)
- Medium- and full-sized trampolines
- Bounce houses
- BOSU balls (domed side up)
- Cushioned mats/spring floors

But beds and other objects are not designed to provide a continuous or rigorous workout, and won't last long even if you do manage to get a good bounce out of them from time to time. Which is why, of course, *the only type of rebounding workout we discuss and recommend is one undertaken on a rebounder* designed as personal exercise equipment.

If you have access to a medium- or full-sized trampoline, it's certainly *possible* to get a good or even great rebounding workout on one. In addition to their size, however, there are some distinct disadvantages to trampolines for the type of health-and-wellness-focused practice discussed here. Let's consider these differences more closely.

Trampolines may, but do not usually, give the same kind of tightly controlled bounce that a rebounder does. On a trampoline large enough for more than one person, it's harder to stay in one place and go through the kind of sequences and powerful patterned repetitions that are typically at the heart of rebounding as an energizing health and fitness practice.

And, on a trampoline, most people are eventually...inevitably...tempted to do at least an occasional gymnastic movement or "stunt" that would be inappropriate for a rebounder.

This is fine if you're interested in doing these kinds of movements—and you know how to stay safe while doing them—but it's quite distinct from what makes rebounding so beneficial and so much fun in the first place. Plus, playing around with stunts can divert you from establishing the Bounce as a regular practice. Moreover, trampolines are not nearly as portable as rebounders. You can't, for example, set them up in your living room to watch TV or listen to music, and you can't easily take them with you on vacation.

But, but, but: Big Trampolines Are So Much Fun!

Yes, exactly! They really *can* be a ton of fun, but ask yourself this: Is it the size of the trampoline that creates that awesome fun feeling, or is it the Bounce itself? Is it the size of the gravity ship that matters, or your personal motion within the gravity ocean?

The fact that you can get most of the same great fun feeling while bouncing on a small personal rebounder as you can on an outdoor trampoline—but have that fun with relatively little danger—is well worth contemplating. With most of the fun, and almost none of the danger, for those interested in establishing a health and fitness practice, rebounders are a really good bet.

We don't want to be spoilsports: trampolines can be great if you like them, you own one, your weather's usually good, and you *want to* be trampolining, including doing stunts. (And you also don't mind the danger—to you or to any children with access.[8]) Still, for as long as we've been working on raising consciousness about rebounding, we've

---

8   According to the Mayo Clinic, "Trampoline jumping poses a high risk of injury for children. The activity can result in sprains and fractures in the arms or legs—as well as potentially serious head and neck injuries.... Trampoline park injuries also are an area of emerging concern." Rebounders are *much* less dangerous than full-sized trampolines. Even so, you'll see an ongoing focus throughout this book on having safety as a # 1 priority for your rebounding practice.

never heard of anyone who has established a regular rebound exercise practice on an outdoor trampoline. You *could* do it, of course, but *why* would you? Unless you're a former gymnast or trampoline athlete, you won't be missing much.

The bottom line is that if you want to truly experience and regularly practice rebound exercise—if you want to maximize the benefits of the Bounce—you'll need to do so on rebound exercise equipment that is designed as such. Compared to a trampoline—even a good one—a quality rebounder provides a safer, more contained, and more convenient experience that's qualitatively different both safety-wise and in the feel of the bouncing experience. And it makes establishing a regular practice much, much easier.

The Evolution of Rebounders and Some Recommended Types and Brands[9]

When Jordan first started bouncing daily[10] at age 42 in 2002, several different brands and types of spring-based rebounders—including some supposedly high-quality ones—simply fell apart under his rigorous usage (for example, when he was doing his first-ever 45 X 45 Challenge outdoors with hand weights). Either the springs broke, the mats frayed and fell apart, or both. Later on, the bellicon company came out with a higher-quality unit whose springs did not break and whose mats did not come apart no matter how "all out" he went. Eventually, bellicon's expensive but very high-quality bungee-based units became available, and now less expensive bungee-based units are also coming to market.

---

9   Many people ask us if we design or sell rebounders. In fact, once upon a time Jordan did sell them, and he also worked briefly with an inventor on a brand-new concept for a lightweight, inexpensive, portable bouncer. For now, though, unless and until we design a rebounder that's distinctly better than what's currently available, we're quite content to stay out of the bouncer business. We leave that to others, and we congratulate them on building better and better rebounders at ever more affordable prices. Our primary passion and goal is to motivate and mentor people on how to *use* the rebounder they already have or decide to obtain. If and when someone comes up with a breakthrough, we'll do our best to let you know as soon as possible.

10   For the record, Jordan first started bouncing on a cheap spring-based rebounder in 1984 when living in a small studio apartment in Astoria, Queens. After about three weeks, he stopped using it forever, and he didn't start bouncing again until a friend brought a high-quality unit to his home in 2002.

What's important to know is that rebounders are overall worlds better than when they first debuted in the late 1970s. (For some context, please see Appendix A, which provides a brief history of rebound exercise overall.) We agree with Al Carter, "the father of rebound exercise" (whose company still provides midrange spring-based rebounders), as to why the initial fad or craze of the 70s and 80s fizzled out: too many low-quality, poorly made copycat rebounders rapidly flooded the market. This led to many unpleasant, unproductive, and even harmful situations. In addition to providing a mediocre and unpleasant bouncing experience, low-quality units can break underneath you as you bounce, or simply fall apart too quickly, rather than providing years of good use.

Fortunately, there have now been several generations of improved equip-ment design. Good-quality beginner- and intermediate-level rebounders are available from several manufacturers. And while as of this writing you can still spend up to $1,000—with tax and delivery—to buy what's probably the best bungee-based rebounder out there (the bellicon), you can also have a safe, enjoyable, healthy, and inspiring rebounding experience on a different bungee-based rebounder for just a little over $200 (from Leaps & Rebounds). Intermediate and high-quality spring- and bungee-based units from manufacturers such as Cellerciser, JumpSport, Needak, and ReboundAir (Al Carter's company) are also available in the United States as of this writing, and we can expect more decent-quality, low-cost bun-gee-based units to follow.

Rebounders are literally full of moving parts, constantly impacted by your bodyweight in motion. It takes quality parts to be able to offer a rebounder that will be safe and pleasant to use, and long lasting. If a rebounder costs too little—for example, less than $100—then it's almost certainly essen-tially a "toy," and you're not nearly as likely to have a positive, productive, and enduring experience. Low-quality units cannot give you the same kind of bounce, and because of their construction, mat quality, spring (or bungee) quality, and so on, they may even aggravate your existing physical conditions rather than help rehabilitate them. Jordan has had people try high quality and inexpensive rebounders side by side many times. No one who has tried both has doubted the value of spending the extra money to obtain a decent-quality rebounder.

Suppose you spend $200 or even go all the way up to $1,000 for a high-quality rebounder. In our view, that's a great deal for equipment that will—potentially for decades[11]—provide you with a daily exercise platform as well as inspiration and delight. The price of a rebounder is clearly a bargain compared to a monthly gym membership, a treadmill or rower, or the price of specialized equipment for just about any other kind of sport, outdoor recreation, or exercise program. Even runners sometimes spend as much in shoes each year as a rebounder costs just once for many years of use.

  Four Rules of Thumb

1. You'll need an actual rebounder to undertake a successful rebound exercise practice; a bed, air mattress, or outdoor trampoline just won't do.

2. Buy the very best rebounder you can afford.

3. Bungee-based rebounders are what most people will be happiest with—they are a tremendous innovation—but there are some exceptions and caveats.

4. Be careful with rebounders with folding frames and mats (that fold in halves thirds, or even worse, quarters). Folding legs are usually OK, based on brand.

Stabilizing or Holding Bars: Only If You Really Need One

A stabilizing or holding bar that attaches to a rebounder is available for many brands. They are usually not that expensive—they typically cost $50 to $100 on top of whatever the bouncer costs—and are relatively easy to install.

---

11   Note that springs can break on spring-based units, and the bands on bungee-based units will eventually wear out and need to be replaced. Any rebounder may eventually need a new mat.

The real question is *whether you need one at all*. Holding on to or leaning on the bar not only bends you over—impeding breathing and contorting your whole body—but makes it very difficult to do many otherwise natural rebounding movements that involve freely moving in all dimensions. Some holding bars attach in such a way that they cut across the mat, drastically limiting your usable mat surface and overall bouncing area. ("Hey, who put that metal railing right through the middle of my Bounce space?")

Admittedly, for young children and the elderly, and others who have very poor balance or are just too unstable or uncertain, a holding bar can provide a big advantage. It can take away the fear of bouncing right off the mat or losing one's balance. Without a bar, some people might not be able to bounce at all.

On the other hand, many people—including those who are at first uncertain or a little bit wobbly—find that their balance rapidly improves after a few bouncing sessions. It often becomes clear that there isn't (and never really was) any need for a holding bar.

If you fall into the first group, then by all means, go ahead and get one. Then, if your balance and confidence improve, you can forgo its use and remove it entirely. Another option is to use a stretchy band threaded under the rebounder's mat, and hold on to both ends of it for help with balance. Finally, you can hold onto high-backed chairs placed on either side of you, or bounce next to a wall and lean on it when necessary.

Handheld Weights, Other Accessories, and Miscellaneous Gear

Bouncing with light handheld weights is invaluable, especially if you want gains in muscle size, tone, and strength, as well as in overall flexibility. Generally, though, you want to keep yourself to *light* weights, or you can strain or otherwise hurt yourself. (While a pair of weights may seem very light—such as pairs of three-, two-, or even one-pound weights—their perceived heaviness and overall effectiveness are multiplied both by their being in motion and by the general precepts of the physics of fitness, which we'll get to later.)

Dr. Harry Sneider and his wife, Sarah, who wrote *Harry and Sarah Sneider's Olympic Trainer: Fitness Excellence through Resistive Rebounding* (2000), developed hand weights filled with sand for rebounding, called "sandbags," that are easy to grip and mold to your hands.

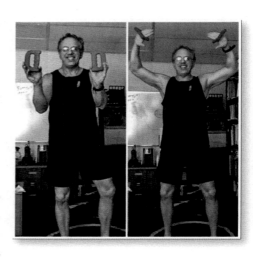

Some people prefer using Velcro-enabled or strap-on weighted gloves, but we like neoprene weights that are soft to hold and cause little damage even if dropped. Plus, handheld weights shaped like the letter "D" offer an interesting advantage.

You can extend your fingers, hands, or wrists through the weight, and then bounce *without* gripping or using your hand or finger strength to actually hold on to it. Through leverage and the physics of fitness, this frees you to more specifically target particular muscle groups, such as those in your back and shoulders. The difference between gripping and not gripping may not seem like much at first, but with many repetitions of a single movement (with variations), it makes a big difference.

Whatever type of handheld weights you get, we recommend you get at least two or three pairs, starting very light and then moving up. A good place to start is with pairs of one-, two-, and three-pound weights—Jordan still uses all three of these weights in his daily bounce—but you can also get, for instance, ones, threes, and fives. The heavier handheld weights are, the more they cost, but none of the lighter-weight pairs (ones, twos, threes, fours, or fives) are all that expensive. And, of course, even if the D-shaped handheld weights are ideal, there's no reason you can't use any light dumbbell pairs you happen to already have.

Some people like to jump rope while bouncing—it's a great aerobic workout and calls for a lot of coordination. You'll need a good jump rope for this. While your childhood one (if you still have it) might be okay, it's worth going to a sporting goods store to check out current models and find one you like that's the right length.

There's not a lot else that you need to get going with rebounding. It may be useful to have a towel to wipe off your body or your feet. As with any exercise, it is always good to have water nearby. And if you're going to bounce outdoors, in the sun, sunscreen and a secure hat may be advisable. If your indoor rebounding space isn't private, lightweight portable headphones will help you enjoy your favorite music (as loud as you like) without disturbing others. Jordan's wireless telephone headset lets him comfortably combine conversations and bounce time—with his mom, friends, and even clients. Finally, if you're going to have your hands busy with weights or jump rope handles, you might want to wear gloves while bouncing.

Shake Weights: An Inexpensive but Invaluable Accessory

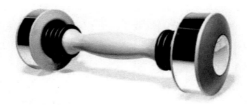

Shake Weights, introduced around 2010 and priced around $20 each, are small handheld dumbbells that internally move or "shake." Based on how they are held, moved, and shaken, they produce novel, challenging, and stimulating feedback. Despite some silly, suggestive, and often-parodied marketing, they're a great addition to any practice of the Bounce, especially if you have a matched pair.

Most people buy only one Shake Weight, but having one for each hand while bouncing is much better. We suggest you buy two of the women's Shake Weights. The men's version is identical, except for weighing twice as much (five pounds each), which makes them much harder to shake or move in any way (especially with one hand). Men and women alike typically find that the lower weight, once it's in motion, is ample for challenging their strength and improving their experience. After learning to shake the weights (while bouncing) with your wrists and arms, you can move the focus of the work to your shoulders and back, which is much more challenging.

Safety Guide: A Bounce of Prevention's Worth a Pound of Cure

You've received your wonderful brand-new rebounder in the mail, or perhaps from a nearby store, and have successfully set it up. (Usually this just means screwing on or unfolding the legs, but you may also have to attach bungee bands or undertake some simple mechanical procedures. Usually no special tools are required, although a hex key, Allen wrench, or other fastening device may come with your rebounder.)

There it sits in front of you, and you're just so excited to get on and try it out. But before you hop on, let's discuss how you can establish a safe and injury-free practice of the Bounce that will potentially serve you for the rest of your life.

By definition, rebounders are spring-loaded—whether they make use of bungee bands or actual springs made of metal or plastic—and almost the entire rest of the world is not. This seems obvious, but once you get on your rebounder and begin bouncing—especially if you're an eager and energetic person—there's a tendency to bounce right off of it. The ground the rebounder is on is never as forgiving as the rebounder itself, and you can seriously injure your ankles or feet if you land incorrectly.

A rebounder is a relatively safe device—for example, it's much more forgiving on the skeleton and joints than running on hard ground could ever be, and you don't have to deal with cars, bikes, weather, potholes, or dogs. But very importantly, it's still potentially dangerous if misused, or used without awareness. Anything with so much potential to transform your life also has the potential—and, for you physics geeks, the harnessed potential energy!—to cause harm if you do not remain safety-focused, aware, and conscious of what you're up to at all times. Treat your rebounder with respect, and you can develop a long, safe, and extremely beneficial relationship with it.

Rebounders are substantial devices or instruments, and rebounding is powerful medicine. Be conscious and alert and follow common sense, and you can prevent yourself and anyone nearby from ever having a rebounding-related injury. Aim to never harm yourself or anyone else while bouncing, that is, aim to *never* have a Bounce-related accident.

While accidents related to rebound exercise *are nearly 100% preventable, it all depends upon you*. So embrace the axiom that safety, just as much as vibrant health, well-being, and even enlightenment itself, starts with awareness. And then make it your sacred vow to personally take responsibility for adding to the ongoing legacy of rebounding safety. Get on and off safely, stop if you need to, don't leave your rebounder out when not in use, and follow all the other safety rules put forth in this book. Yes, all of them.

Your Physician's Approval:
Do you Need It/Can (Should) You Override it?

Before even stepping onto a rebounder, you may want to have an expert make sure you're physically qualified for bouncing. Generally, before undertaking any new—or resuming any old—physical exercise or practice, you should begin by thoroughly evaluating your own condition. And if you have any concerns, or any active disabilities or medical conditions requiring treatment, you should seek the advice of a medical professional. This is as true for rebounding as it is for any potentially vigorous exercise program.

Don't be fooled by the apparent gentleness of rebound exercise or the fact that it's truthfully promoted throughout this book as being "fun and easy." It can be gentle, fun, and easy; it also can be very physically challenging and demanding. The simple rule of thumb here is this:

If rebounding worsens an existing physical injury or limitation, or if your doctor or other healthcare provider forbids you from rebounding, then don't.

Since no license or prescription is needed to buy a rebounder and step onto it, it's up to you, personally, to honestly and seriously evaluate whether you need to first see a physician or other qualified healthcare giver. If you're young and healthy, you might not need to worry very much about this. But everyone else should soberly and carefully evaluate their overall health, as well as any particular limiting physical conditions they may have, before starting or intensifying a rebounding practice.

Unfortunately, there are some people for whom rebounding is simply not physically appropriate. For example, if you have a ruptured or herniated spinal disc condition, or if you have a serious (chronic or acute) knee, foot, or ankle injury, then you may not be able to engage in the Bounce. In fact, if you have any serious physical disability or preexisting condition, be prepared for a competent and qualified physician (or other healthcare provider) to indeed declare the Bounce off limits for you.

Still, many people—including those with injuries, lower back problems, or just the need to tone up and get into shape—will find themselves wondering whether rebounding can benefit them. Let's take a step back and remember that a good rebounder will absorb about five-sixths of the physical shock to the body that comes from exercising at the same exertion level on hard non-giving ground. This means two things.

First, bouncing is a good and often great alternative for those who like aerobic exercise but may have incurred bone, joint, or connective tissue damage from running, jogging, racquet sports, basketball, dancing, skiing, martial arts, or just day-to-day life. As you read through promotional materials for rebound exercise or specific rebounder brands, you'll often find the low-impact nature of bouncing called out, and rightly so. For example, if you love to run but no longer can...well, with a good bouncer, you just might be able to run again as much as you like, albeit in place.

Second, it's important to follow your intuition when conventional medical authorities say you probably shouldn't be bouncing. In some cases, these will be exactly the kinds of conditions that rebounding *might actually be best able to help with*. For example, if you suffer from lower back pain, the rebounder's ability to strengthen abdominal muscles may help that pain.

Or if you have knee problems, a quality bouncer absorbs a great deal of the impact while nonetheless giving you (including your knees) a thorough workout that may help heal that pain. In fact, both the creator of Urban Rebounding™, J.B. Berns, and Jordan's IP attorney, who helped with Super-Bound®, rehabilitated their knees through bouncing. (The key is to go slowly and be very careful of exactly how much weight you put on the troubled knee and what you ask it to do.)

There are few cut-and-dried rules here. For some people, any kind of existing pain that might be stimulated, re-stimulated, or "pushed to its edges" through bouncing's repetitive motion might disqualify them from rebounding. For others, the many positive known and suspected healing and energizing qualities of the rebounder will more than outweigh that risk, even if there is some pain ("good pain") involved at first. Joy's personal experience is instructive (note that in the adjacent photo, she is in her early 60s):

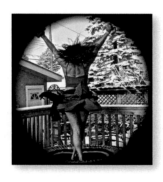

> You may be surprised to learn that I have a history of ongoing back pain. When people watch our SuperBound bounce videos, I look (and feel) more like a limber 40-year-old than an over-60 woman with some significant physical challenges. After my back was severely injured over a decade ago—MRIs showed my lower vertebrae were a compacted utter mess—I was unable to walk for close to a full month. This was terrifying, as I love to dance—I've been a dancer all my life!—and the thought I might never be able to dance again was absolutely shattering.
>
> I slowly healed, but my back wasn't really getting all the way better. Regardless of how careful I was, I regularly experienced my back "going out" on me. My legs would also go numb, or else sometimes hurt so much I could barely walk. In addition to my sciatica issues, arthritis runs in my family (my dad was crippled by it in his early 60s), and X-rays showed arthritis in my hips. I've also experienced knee pain, especially when walking up too many stairs.

All of these conditions and their associated pain have changed so much for the better over my now many years of regular rebounder use! My back and knees have strengthened remarkably, and overall my regular practice of the Bounce has proven remarkably effective physical therapy for me. I hate to imagine how physically awful I'd likely still feel from all conditions if I hadn't been so dedicated to my rebounding practice!

Classic back relief exercises did help a little, but nothing, absolutely nothing, helped me and still helps me as powerfully as does regular bouncing. Just keep in mind you need to start very slow and gentle. Begin with simply standing on your rebounder mat and moving back and forth with conscious care. If you feel any discomfort, shift your weight gently in different directions until you find the "sweet spot" where you can move without pain. Over time you should find those areas improve in mobility, flexibility, and strength. Among other things, a rebounder really is a leveraged platform for healing.

Although the relationship between physical movement itself and healing is not completely understood, it's clear to us that in some cases it's nothing more than the regular movement of the body on the rebounder that brings about healing. For example, about 15 years ago, Jordan was able to work through and heal long-standing and worsening pain from a torn rotator cuff by doing 100 arm circles in both directions while bouncing—over a period of only two months. Yes, it was a little uncomfortable at first, but as he stayed present with his breath and his sensations, it didn't take long for the healing to kick in.

If every doctor you see, including alternative practitioners, tells you that rebounding is not a good idea for you, then you just may not be able to go forward with it. But if you get a variety of professional opinions, you should carefully weigh the choices before you.

Just don't sell yourself short: many believe that rebound exercise can speed the rehabilitation of muscle and joint injuries. If you work with your breath and go slow and easy, bouncing may be helpful with both rehabilitation and pain relief.

The Physical Setting

The location where you bounce can make a big difference to your rebound exercise experience. Wherever you intend to rebound, ask yourself the following safety questions:

- Is the surface I'm going to bounce on reasonably flat and level?
- Can the surface I bounce on, and any structure attached to it, withstand the force of vigorous rebounding?
- Will a rug—or any other soft or finished indoor or outdoor surface— be damaged or permanently marked (with round depressions) by the rebounder's legs?
- Do I have enough room above and around me? (Extend your arms fully and see if they hit the ceiling or any objects to the side of you.)

The bottom line is that you need enough room to be able to fully extend your arms out sideways, as well as fully over your head while you're in mid-bounce, and you need a level floor and structure that can handle the force of bouncing. You may have a perfect place in your home, indoors or outdoors, for bouncing but have unfettered access to it only for a limited time each day. Be wise, be crafty, and be persistent, and the right opportunity for you to bounce will show up each day.

If your space isn't big enough for you to "bounce big," then don't. If you're in a place with low ceilings, bounce lower! The same thing applies to walls, furniture, or objects that might be in your way: avoid them! Save your "big bouncing" for outdoors or when you have more room indoors. Hint: you can keep your arms low in ceiling-challenged spaces; if it's such a low space that your head will hit the ceiling, then keep your feet—and even your heels—on the mat.

With respect to carpets, most quality carpets are able to withstand the round depressions potentially made by the force of bouncing transmitted through the rebounder's legs. There have been times, however, especially when bouncing in other people's homes, when we have stuck folded pieces of thick paper or cardboard under each of the legs to avoid any possibility of permanent damage. Certain types of coasters can also be used, but can break if they're too rigid or brittle.

Finally, when bouncing indoors, *be especially careful about objects potentially toppling over* (like pieces of furniture or large home theater units), or small objects that slowly but surely vibrate over to the edge of shelves and bookcases and then crash to the floor. You can usually tell pretty quickly which objects are problematic, but sometimes it helps to have someone who isn't bouncing give you a stable third-party perspective.

Bouncing Outdoors: We enthusiastically recommend bouncing outdoors, at least from time to time, when you have the opportunity. As with most athletic activities, people report bouncing "bigger," "higher," and more vigorously outdoors.

Bouncing in Private: Whether to bounce around others is a personal decision. Some people really don't mind having others around. Rebounding can make a great social activity: Joy and Jordan both like bouncing around other people. But many folks strongly prefer bouncing alone, and that's just fine.

Ultimately, where to bounce comes down to what you prefer and what's available. Try to find someplace in or around your home that usually works, and then look for a few alternative locations to spice things up when you have the opportunity.

Bouncing on the Road: Travel and Vacation

Joy and Jordan both like rebounding in novel venues—that is, wherever it is they happen to be when traveling or on vacation. Yes, it can be a bit of an effort to bring along a rebounder, but for those who don't like going more than a few days without bouncing—especially when subjected to the stresses of travel—it's well worth it to bring one along (especially on car trips; it's not so easy if you're flying).

Rebounding has multiple travel-specific benefits. First, it stimulates the digestive system to keep elimination on track. Second, it boosts your illness-fighting immune system. This is particularly beneficial for those who sleep poorly on the road, and for everyone who has to deal with the increased germ exposure that inevitably accompanies travel.

Note, however, that it's very important to make sure that whatever building or structure you're rebounding in can handle the force that is transmitted through the rebounder legs into the floor! Once, while on a family vacation in Mendocino, California, in a rented cabin right on the coast, Jordan put his rebounder on the second floor and began bouncing. A couple of minutes later a family member came racing up the stairs shouting that the whole house was shaking and might collapse! Jordan adapted, bouncing lower and slower inside, and then outside whenever he could for the remainder of the vacation.

Mat, Springs/Bands, Legs:
Your Rebounder's Pre-Session Safety Checklist

Don't rebound if your rebounder is substantially damaged in any way. Before every rebounding session, you should check to make sure that your bouncer is in good working condition and ready to go. Here are some things to look for:

- If you have a folding rebounder, is it fully unfolded and locked into position?
- Are all of your rebounder's legs fully down and in their locked position? Or if your rebounder has screw-on legs, are they fully and securely screwed on, with a locking pin or wire in place if that's part of the leg design?
- Is the mat in good condition? Make sure it's not substantially frayed, coming apart at the edges where it is sewed on, or otherwise damaged.
- Are all of your springs or bungee bands in good shape? If you have one spring that is damaged or a bit bent out of shape, you can still bounce, but you should replace that spring as soon as possible—call the manufacturer for replacements. Even one bad spring will immediately start putting uneven stress, wear, and tear on the rest

of the rebounder. On bungee-based units, if an individual bungee band breaks, you should stop bouncing and replace it (or, better yet, replace the whole set because they'll probably start breaking like popcorn, one by one, especially whenever you really get going and start bouncing more intensely).

- If there is a spring cover, is it caught on a hinge or tangled up in the springs?
- Is the mat dry, and is there an absence of debris?

In some situations, like bouncing outdoors when it's windy, debris from plants, trees, and other sources can accumulate on your rebounder even in the middle of a bounce session. The easiest way to get the debris off is with a small brush (a whisk brush is perfect) or a towel (you can whip-snap with a towel or shirt and usually clear the bouncer in one or two shots). There are times when you'll want to stop your workout, step off the bouncer, turn it on its side, and lightly tap it with your fingers to remove the debris. You may also be tempted to get little pieces of debris and grit off your feet *while* you're bouncing, but this is generally not a good idea. Even if you have to break your rhythm, you're better off stopping to brush it off, since doing so is both more effective and far safer.

Know When (and How) to Fold 'Em

Be careful when folding a folding rebounder. Follow the manufacturer's instructions exactly, or injury can result.

Some rebounders have split frames that let them be folded up for compact storage and travel. If your rebounder folds into halves, thirds, or even fourths, carefully follow the manufacturer's instructions on folding and unfolding. One unit we tested—a "quarterfold" that folded twice down the middle!—had such high tension on the springs that two people were needed to safely work with it. Other units, especially half-folds, are under much less tension and can usually safely be folded by one person.

Be especially careful with your face, fingers, toes, jewelry, rugs and carpets, spring (or bungee) covers, and anything else that can get caught as you close a folding rebounder (including pets and children). And always remember that these units can snap open with quite a bit of force, so be careful to clear the area first. Try to open a folding rebounder on a soft surface such as a rug, carpet, or patch of grass.

Lastly, over time the hinges on folding rebounders can loosen up some, so be careful when you're moving a rebounder about that it doesn't suddenly, unexpectedly, and inconveniently fold of its own accord.

While some rebounders have legs that can be folded flat, it's usually easier and more convenient for your next rebounding session if you store the unit on its side, legs fully extended. If you store your rebounder like this, be careful that it is firmly placed and won't slip down, roll away, or topple over. The best solution is a permanent indoor storage space where you can leave the rebounder ready for your next session. While rebounders can be stored outdoors and may be somewhat waterproof, it's much better to not leave them exposed to too much weather, especially rain, snow, and direct sun. The better you treat it, the longer it will last (which in turn will help you last longer!).

After a while you'll be able to tell if your rebounder is ready to go in about 15 seconds or less, but don't be tempted to overlook those 15 seconds!

Starting and Stopping (Mounting and Dismounting) and (Not) Falling Off

Always be careful when getting on or off a rebounder. By definition, rebounders are "spring loaded" (even if they use bungee bands), so when you first step onto one, you want to make sure you don't bounce right off of it. Similarly, you should pretty much stop bouncing completely before you gently step off. It's all too easy to forget that hard ground (even if it is carpeted) does not give the way a rebounder does!

So: *always* pay attention when getting on and getting off a rebounder. Do not leap onto one, and *be especially careful not to leap off of one*! In particular, don't leap off to respond to your phone or the doorbell. Also be careful about your feet and toes when getting on or off: don't become tangled in the bungee bands or, worse, cut by the springs, or otherwise run afoul of either a spring cover or a bungee cover.

As for falling off generally, the good news is that almost everyone who consistently bounces with attention quickly finds that their balance—along with their proprioceptive awareness and general bodily awareness—rapidly improves to the point where they rarely if ever fall off. The one exception to this, which we'll discuss shortly, is that sometimes when bouncing very rapidly or forcefully (e.g., running fast in place with knees going high), it's possible to experience a kind of "glitch" where your smooth movement is interrupted and it feels like you could fall or bounce off.

Additional Safety Factors

Food and Water: Stay adequately hydrated and maintain an adequate blood sugar level, before and during bouncing. Do not bounce when drinking alcohol, and do not eat or drink while bouncing. Don't rebound on a full stomach.

Don't Bounce Dizzy or Inebriated: Do not rebound if you're dizzy, drunk, or otherwise so intoxicated that you might fall off or hurt yourself.

Children and Pets: Watch out for children and pets while bouncing. Be aware of animals—especially dogs and some cats—who may try to get on the rebounder with you. It's all too easy to have your balance thrown off (which can lead to you falling off) if another being (human or animal) hops onto your rebounder while you're bouncing.

Kids love bouncing and are very attracted to it. They also usually want to do stunts, bounce as high as they can (and then right off the rebounder), and get on the mat at the same time as their friend(s). Generally, it's recommended that you not let any young children (under 12) bounce alone, because they will inevitably drift toward unsafe movement or start leaping onto and off of the mat. Even older children should not be left to bounce unsupervised, unless in your judgment the child in question is mature enough to understand and respect the rebounder and always act safely on and around it. Letting older children supervise younger children is generally not a good idea, unless you have absolute faith in the constant alertness and good judgment of the older child.

The Elderly and Infirm: As for elderly and infirm individuals, as previously discussed you can buy a stabilizing bar that fits onto the legs or frame of the bouncer to provide a place to hold on to. For some people, it is simply impossible to bounce without a stabilizing bar. Note that if someone does need a stabilizing bar, it's usually a good idea to have someone else there to help them on and off and monitor them, at least at first. Another option for the elderly and infirm is what's called a "bounce back chair." After you sit in the seat of the chair—which is attached to a tall metal frame by long springs—you can push off with whatever arm or leg strength you have to bring about a nice smooth bouncing motion, along with all of the benefits that provides.

Pain: Whatever your age, if you have any pain, listen to it, and if it continues, stop bouncing. Common sense is always the best guide: if something hurts, stop bouncing; if you're dizzy, stop bouncing; if the rebounder or the location where you're bouncing is problematic, then stop bouncing immediately.

Too Heavy? Don't bounce on a rebounder if you outweigh its poundage rating. Most quality rebounders are rated at 250 or 300 pounds, and some are rated at 400 pounds. All quality rebounders have a recommended weight range, and certain brands and model types are noted for having a softer bounce, a springier bounce, or something in between. If nothing else, there will be a maximum weight limit that you should not go over.

If you're near the top end of the poundage rating and you bounce long and vigorously, you may find that your rebounder's parts, especially the mats and springs or bungees, wear out faster than you'd originally hoped for. Also, even those who weigh much less than 300 pounds may find that with very vigorous bouncing, certain foot positions (such as landing on your heels) can lead to "bottoming out" or having your heels hit the floor through the rebounder's mat at the very bottom of your up-and-down cycle.

Exactly Where on the Rebounder to Bounce (the Mat) and Where Not To: During active rebound exercise sessions, you might move your body and feet all the way around the mat, turning in all directions. On occasion, you may find that you've bounced on the stitched outer ring, on the spring (or bungee) cover, or even right on a spring or bungee. This typically won't hurt you or the rebounder too badly, although bouncing on a spring can be painful, and if your feet get tangled up in the springs, bungees, or spring/bungee cover, you can fall and substantially hurt yourself. In any case, always get back to bouncing in "fair territory" as soon as possible.

Think of it this way: you should bounce on your rebounder in the way it was designed to be bounced on, i.e., only in "fair territory." So bounce anywhere you want on the mat itself, but try *not* to bounce on the springs or bungee bands, the spring or bungee cover (if your rebounder has one), or the rebounder's frame. Only the mat is designed to provide a flexible, resilient surface suitable for bouncing.

Warm-ups and Cool Downs: As a general principle, as with other types of exercise, it's important to warm up and cool down to prevent injury and mobilize your physical and energetic resources. On the one hand, you can bounce very slowly at first to get a kind of warm-up in on the rebounder. But if you have done other sports and physical activities and have a way of stretching or warming up that you know works for you, we recommend that you take advantage of it. While some folks have put together entire warm-up routines that you can do *while* on your rebounder, there's no real need for this. Instead, this is one of those things that you can figure out for yourself—and that will work better for you when you've done so.

As for cool downs, everything we said about warm-ups applies to them as well. You know what you need to do. Most of us will want to slow down our bouncing as we near the end of our practice time, and if it's helpful for you, go ahead and stretch some (particularly quads, hamstrings, and so on).

Don't Sweat a Glitch or a Hitch: Sometimes, when bouncing forcefully or at a rapid rate (e.g., running fast in place with knees very high), it's possible to experience a kind of "glitch" where your smooth movement becomes interrupted and it feels like you could fall or bounce off. This can also be thought of as a hitch in your stride, or as if you were a guitar string that had been plucked and "twanged" in precisely the wrong way at precisely the wrong moment.

It can feel pretty bad when this happens. Essentially, our bodies some-times let go of tension in funny ways that feel almost worse than the tension itself. In any case, you'll definitely know it when you feel it.

If this kind of glitch should happen to you, simply adjust your style of bouncing—the movements, the patterns, the pace—and keep on going. If you stay aware and don't worry or panic, you'll probably be able to continue with your workout just fine. That is, continue with your rebounding session gently and with awareness. Just make sure you didn't injure yourself, and give some loving attention and apply whatever healing knowledge and tools you have to the affected area or muscle.

Don't Get Distracted: Watch out for pets, children, and other mid-session distractions (including electronic ones). If something happens in the real world that needs your full attention, then safely get off your rebounder to deal with it. Don't try to address a significant distraction while you're still bouncing, as that can be dangerous.

Limit Small Screens: This is, of course, just a subset of "Don't Get Dis-tracted." Be very careful about—and whenever possible avoid using—cell phones or other "screens" while bouncing. The email, the text, the update, whatever it is…can and should wait.

Stay in Control: Don't bounce too much or too intensely, especially at first. Don't start out too quickly; moderate your intensity, as well as total bounce time, for your first few rebounding sessions and, for that matter, your first few weeks. Don't bounce so high that you tend to bounce off the rebounder or lose control. Always be safe.

One at a Time, and No Stunts! Don't allow two or more people to bounce on one rebounder at the same time. Rebounders are not designed for this, and harm can result.

How about doing some simple stunts on rebounders or doubles bounc-ing? Just a few seat drops, perhaps? No, no, no! Again, rebounders are descended from but are *not* mini-trampolines. They are *not* designed for any kind of stunts, not even seat drops, and you should never do stunts or allow others, especially children, to do stunts on rebounders.

Don't Turn Your Bouncer Into a Low-Slung Hazard (Especially in the Dark): A rebounder is a substantial physical object. If you leave one where it isn't expected, it can become a substantial hazard. Since most rebounders are eight to 14 inches off the ground, they can easily be missed and trip an unsuspecting person. So please do not leave your rebounder on the ground where it doesn't belong, especially outdoors at night, or in any dark or potentially dark place.

When Jordan first obtained a decent-quality rebounder in 2002, he was so excited about having it and wanting others to try it that he left it outside on his deck. His journal entry reads: "I promptly forgot that I had left it outside on the ground, and when darkness came I tripped over it, went flying, and hit the ground. I could have seriously injured myself, and feel very lucky I escaped with just a scrape or two. So even if you think you'll be coming back in just a few minutes, *don't* leave your rebounder in a place where it might pose a danger if you happen to forget about it. It's just not worth the risk."

Two Legs Good! *(At Least for a Year).* Bouncing on a rebounder with just one leg can be pretty difficult, especially at first. We went back and forth several times about whether to include one-legged bouncing in this book at all. Ultimately, we decided that instruction on one-legged bouncing is best saved for our next set of more advanced materials. Even Jordan, who has been bouncing now for close to 20 years, finds one-legged bouncing pretty challenging and demanding. So our advice is this: don't even think about trying one-legged bouncing until you have at least a year of regular bouncing behind you. It's just too easy for things to go wrong, and as always, safety comes first.

Setting Up and Getting Ready

Socks and Shoes: Not Recommended Unless Really Needed

Should you bounce with or without socks and shoes? Both of your authors have a strong personal preference for bouncing *without*, and therefore almost never do so. Bouncing without socks and shoes gives your bare feet and toes the freedom and flexibility to explore subtle differences that come from, for example, angling your feet slightly differently, or putting pressure more on the insides versus the outsides of your feet, or putting more weight on the heels versus the toes versus the balls of the feet, and so on. If you're wearing socks and shoes, you generally won't be aware of these dynamics, nor will you be able to do much about them.

So unless there's a good reason to do otherwise—and there are a couple of those—we recommend bouncing *without* socks and shoes. We believe you'll be far better off having your bare feet interacting directly with the mat. Doing so gives you a better feel for the rebounder, and over time will enable you to do far more work with all 26 of the fine bones in your feet, as well as with your ankles, lower legs, and so on. Put differently, socks and especially shoes keep your feet from fully spreading out and feeling the mat, which hinders proprioceptive mechanisms and signal pathways that resonate throughout your body and back to your brain—and you don't want that, do you?

Of course, if it's cold where you're bouncing or if for some reason your rebounder mat is slippery, then you might want socks and shoes. Similarly, if you need special support shoes for orthopedic or other medical reasons, then of course you should wear whatever is necessary and appropriate. And if you're in a gym environment, where many people use the same rebounder—or even in a home environment where there are multiple people bouncing—it should be regularly wiped down and disinfected, whatever footwear might be used.

While you can wear socks and shoes if you really want to,[12] our view remains that our incredible feet deserve to be fully deployed, used, and loved through the bouncing process, and that anyone who doesn't bounce barefoot (if they can) is missing a lot. We suggest you try it out for yourself. Do 10 minutes with your shoes and socks on, and 10 minutes with them off. See which way feels better to you and gives you a better bounce, and we're confident you'll make the right choice.

---

12   If you *are* going to bounce with shoes, then make sure that they are not the type that will rip the mat. No cleats, heavy boots, or high heels! If you need foot or ankle support, we recommend wrapping your ankle or wearing a brace that you can safely move in.

Clothing: What to Wear When You're Both Up and Down

What type of clothing is best for bouncing? To make rebound exercise as fun and easy as possible, you want as few obstacles in the way as possible. Clothing that binds, is too tight, or that otherwise constricts your movement in any way should be avoided.

Generally, then, you want to wear loose, comfortable clothing. You don't want to be cold, but bouncing can also generate a lot of heat. As usual, layers are best. If it's warm enough (outdoors or indoors), you can bounce in shorts and short sleeves, and men may want to bounce shirtless. Many women prefer to wear a sports bra or another supporting garment on top, and some men like to wear support below. If you're bouncing outdoors, depending on the weather you might want socks, long pants, and even a sweatshirt.

We suggest natural fabrics, especially cotton. If you bounce vigorously, you may sweat, so make sure you wear whatever's most comfortable for you. Once again, use what you already know about other sports and activities to make sure that the clothing you wear while rebounding is essentially a nonissue. Of course, if you find a gym with rebounding classes and you care how you look in public, that's a whole 'nother story!

Listening to Music: A Sound Way to Make You Smile and Move

Two of the easiest ways to make sure you get in your daily bouncing time are listening to music (our personal favorite) and watching television.

If you like bouncing with music, then you might want to check with your household members or neighbors and make sure that you're not bothering anyone by turning the music up too loud, either indoors or outdoors. Jordan remarks, "In my household we reached a compromise: I bought a pair of light wireless headphones that I wear to listen to music when other people are at home and not in the mood to share my sonic space."

The same holds for watching TV. Make sure that everyone else is fine with you having it on loudly enough to hear while you bounce, or watch it while you're alone. This advice isn't actually about rebounding specifically; it's simply common sense for shared spaces.

Jordan has found a lightweight cordless headset to also be a good solution for those who like to talk on the telephone while bouncing.

Fitting in the Bounce: Any Time's a Good Time!

The physical benefits associated with bouncing might sound wonderful, but obviously you have to find the time to bounce to actually experience them. How hard is that to do?

One of the Bounce's superpowers is its amazing flexibility when it comes to fitting into your existing timeframe and opportunity set. You can bounce a little bit a few times a day, you can bounce for one or more longer sets, and you can bounce while you're doing other things and still receive tremendous benefits. That is, with the Bounce, your extra "me time" can include TV time, conversations (usually on the phone) with others, or (our favorite) listening to whatever music you most enjoy. The point is that you can often easily layer bouncing on top of other things you find inherently fun and pleasurable, and still receive many of the benefits of the Bounce.

Still, things tend to go better if you plan for them. For example, you don't want to exert yourself and exercise too intensely right after a heavy meal. This is standard advice that we completely support, as bouncing does tend to activate the digestive and eliminative systems. So while this may be more of a "where" than a "when" issue, please be aware that you may need to go to the bathroom—quickly—at a certain point during your daily bounce sessions. Having to urinate about 10 minutes after you start bouncing is not uncommon (which we'll discuss more in chapter 7), and sometimes more than urination will be called for! If you have to interrupt your bouncing routine to take care of personal needs, that's fine. Just get back on the rebounder as soon as you're ready.

Some people like to exercise early in the morning, others later in the evening. Everyone has their own cycle, with some of us more lark-like and others more owl-like. If you do prefer early in the day, make sure your body is sufficiently warmed up. Take a shower or bath or do some other physical activity (like stretching or walking), or just go nice and slow during the beginning of your workout. In other words, it's perfectly fine to warm up on the rebounder itself, especially if you do some of the "Breathwork Bouncing" and "Bodywork Bouncing" we discuss in the next chapter.

How Long Should You Aim to Bounce For at One Time?

Really, it's up to you. But if you want to give yourself the opportunity to receive the greatest possible value from rebound exercise, you should get yourself to the point where you are bouncing for no less than 15 to 30 minutes a day, at least four or five times a week. Obviously, bouncing daily is even better.[13]

We recommend that beginners start with five minutes per session or less. Every few days, add in a few more minutes. You can have multiple bouncing sessions in a day, or take a short break and have another session soon after. One older friend of ours keeps his rebounder out in his living room, and every time he walks by it he gets on for about two minutes. Using a rebounder like this is very different from undertaking rebounding as a focused athletic or transformational activity, but it will nonetheless provide basic immune system, aerobic, stress reduction, and dose-of-daily-fun benefits.

Exercise books often recommend establishing a regular time for your workouts. For some people this does indeed work best. If this suits you, identify a time of the day when you're usually or almost always free, and then set aside at least enough time for your minimum daily session. In this way, you and your body will soon grow used to your regularly scheduled bounce, and even come to expect it at that time of day or night.

If this method works for you, great. But for many people, life is more chaotic than that, and rebounding, like everything else, will have to fit in when it can. But don't make the mistake of waiting until the end of the day

---

13   If that seems like a lot, remember (a) you can do it while watching TV, listening to music, or talking on the phone (especially with wireless earbuds or a headset), and (b) you'll get sick less, you'll become stronger, and your aerobic capacity, balance, and flexibility will all improve. That's worth 15 to 30 minutes a day while you're having fun, isn't it?

and then being too tired. Make rebounding a priority, at least during your initial explorations, so that you can see for yourself whether bouncing daily actually provides the benefits described in this book. Be empirical, and be disciplined. Once you get to experience what rebounding can do for you, it will become easier and easier to make sure you fit it in every day or nearly every day.

There are times when it's nice to not have any time limits—especially when you're feeling good, the environment is the way you like it, and you're free to just let yourself bounce as long as you want. When you're in this sort of "flow" or "bounce trance," time can pass by extremely quickly and pleasantly. And if you gravitate to any of the inner work approaches we'll discuss later, and your rebounding and meditation or other inner work become one and the same, it may be appropriate to bounce for even longer.

A good solid workout—covering aerobic fitness, lymph movement, breath work, and some muscle toning—can be done in a half hour. Half an hour is also, of course, the amount of time that a typical TV program takes, and for those who like to keep up with their favorite shows, a daily dose of bouncing while watching TV is a great way to go.

The bottom line is that you want to bounce when and where you can, for as long as you like, but try to get in at least 10 to 15 minutes a day, and even better is to build up to a half hour or more. If you have any trouble imagining that you can make this work, just remind yourself that there's absolutely nothing more valuable than your health, there's no better way to maintain your health than to have a strong immune system, and rebounding is one of the best means ever invented to accomplish just that.

"But, But...How Do I Actually Start Bouncing?"

How does one actually begin bouncing? This might seem like an odd question. Isn't rebounding itself so simple that it needs no explanation? Or is the act of bouncing inherently so complex and nuanced that it reasonably requires some explanation? The answer is: both. On the one hand, it's absolutely true that you don't really need any instruction on how to actually bounce. Just get on your rebounder and start moving your body. Bend your knees slightly and start rocking back and forth, or push gently down from your core through your feet, and you will indeed begin to bounce up and down.

Whether some or all of both of your feet (and therefore you) leaves the mat entirely depends on how much force you use, so you can play with this a little while to see what it feels like. You can bounce with all of both feet on the mat, with just your heels retaining contact, or in an entirely airborne way (even if it's only a few inches off the mat). Higher is not necessarily better. While there are certain benefits from rebounding that are likely increased by having more "air time" or bouncing higher, doing so also increases the risk of injury. Also, it bears repeating that you can have a totally invigorating, aerobically challenging, muscle- and strength-building, balance-enhancing rebound exercise practice in which your feet never, or rarely, leave the mat.

Now, add in your arms. Move them however you like: up and down, around in circles, flap like a bird, or make swimmer's arms. Guess what? You're successfully rebounding! It couldn't be simpler. Rebounding is all about what feels good to your body, not an artificial set of movements that you enforce upon yourself or copy from others (although that can work too!).

The SuperBound Project always encourages you to find what feels right for your body, mind, and spirit, which may be—and probably is—substantially different than what anyone else needs. That is, your rebounding practice is (and should be) as unique as you and your needs are. Having said that, learning about different ways of bouncing and establishing a successful rebound exercise practice can save you time, spark your creativity, and get you going more quickly.[14] Which brings us to next chapter's "Illustrated Compendium of Bounce Types and Movements."

---

14   If you happen to be a creative cook, reading recipes is a good way to get ideas of how to prepare your next meal, even if you don't follow the recipe to the letter. It's much like that with rebound exercise, that is, reading about—or watching video material on—particular bouncing movements and patterns can inspire you to try something new and wonderful that you might just really love and benefit from.

Section II:

Bounce Ho!

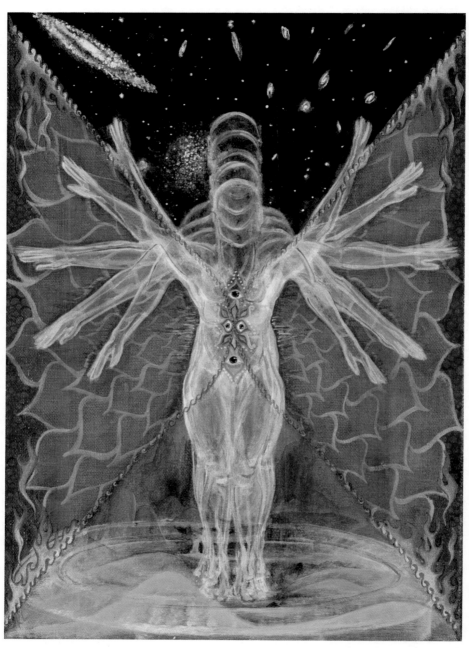

"Cosmic Bound" by Krisztina Lazar

Chapter 5:

An Illustrated Compendium of Bounce Types and Movements

We're big believers in "do your own thing" when it comes to the Bounce. Sure, if you like following along to real world or online bouncing classes, then by all means enjoy! But at the end of the day, at the beginning of the day, and all throughout your day, you'll want to be able to effortlessly move right into your own rebounding practice whenever you feel called. This means you'll want to have thought through, practiced, and established a repertoire of movements and types of bounce that work for you—that you'll commit to and continue with, and that are consistently fun and stimulating.

This chapter provides many ideas for, and illustrations of, different kinds of bounces and movements. Using updated 21st-century terminology, we'll briefly describe the different categories of rebound exercise movements as we see them. Then we'll use these updated categories to describe and illustrate a wide variety of specific bounces and movements.

Taking a step back, one way of framing the development of a personal bouncing practice is to see it as moving through the following stages:

- **Natural Movements** (what you naturally and automatically do on a rebounder, movements that you can and must discover on your own) →
- **Basic Bounces** (which you can either create from your own Natural Movements or draw from the Basic Bounces we describe below) →
- **Simple Routines** (reinforced, amped up, and made super fun by your favorite music, if you're so inclined) →
- **Advanced Routines** (you build these on to your Simple Routines by layering in Expanded Bounces and then Advanced and Specialized Bounces)

Start slow, build up steadily, and before you know it, you'll have your own unique rebound exercise practice that will last you a lifetime!

Three Bounce Type Categories: Our Updated Terminology

Rebound exercise as we know it goes back to the mid-1970s. Since that time, a certain set of terms to describe different types of bounces has been used—and repeated over and over again—in nearly every book written on rebounding. This older terminology is in some ways useful, but in other ways lacking and confusing.[15]

So we've come up with some new terminology that we feel makes more sense and will be more effective in helping you get started with your own Bounce practice. (If you are curious about the older terminology and the problems with it, please see Appendix B.)

Our new terminology is designed to make it easier for everyone to productively discuss rebounding, and to give people who are new to rebound exercise an idea of the wide variety of safe and productive bounces and other movements that are possible. Our three types or major categories of bounces, and the subcategories within them, are:

---

15   The three main terms from the older set of terminology, developed by Al Carter and taken up by almost all subsequent authors, are the "health bounce," roughly equivalent to our Type 1 Easy Bouncing; the "strength bounce," roughly equivalent to our Type 2 High Bouncing; and the "aerobic bounce," roughly equivalent to our Type 2 Fast Bouncing and Running in Place. See Appendix B.

Type 1: Basic Bounces—Simple, Easy Bounces You Can Always Come Back To

    A.   Easy Bouncing (Slow, Low, and Easy)
    B.   Breathwork Bouncing
    C.   Bodywork Bouncing
    D.   Flow Bouncing (Going-with-the-Flow Bouncing)

Type 2: Expanded Bounces—Intermediate and Accessory-Based Bounces

    A.   Bouncing with Handheld Weights, Gloves, and Other Accessories
    B.   Fast Bouncing and Running in Place
    C.   High Bouncing
    D.   Slow Bouncing

Type 3: Advanced and Specialized Bounces

    A.   Cross-Legged Bouncing
    B.   Structured Strength in Motion™ Bouncing
    C.   Abdominal and Stretch Bouncing
    D.   A Cautionary Note on One-Legged Bouncing

Note that each of the main Bounce types has four subcategories within it. In the rest of this chapter we'll go into detail about each type and its subcategories.

Type 1: Basic Bounce—Simple Easy Ones You Can Always Come Back To

A. Easy Bouncing: Slow, Low, and Easy

Rebounding is a fun and easy path to vibrant health and well-being. In fact, to a great extent, it's the very ease we bring to rebounding that makes it so effective. This is true for rebounding both as a health and fitness practice generally and as an activity that can simply and regularly be returned to day after day, month after month, and year after year.

Always remember that even the easiest and simplest ways of moving on a rebounder—keeping it slow, keeping it low, and just keeping it easy overall—will likely bring you substantial health and wellness benefits...that is, as long as you actually keep getting on the mat and moving your body!

In short, while you can always make your rebounding workouts as intense as you like, you can also keep them quite simple, relaxed, and easy while still substantially benefiting. Easy Bouncing movements can be used at any time during a rebounding workout, but are especially good for warming up and cooling down.

The three Easy Bouncing examples (plus variations) are:

1. Pulsing in Place
2. Alternate Feet Shuffle
3. Legs and Feet Twist

Easy Bouncing # 1: Pulsing in Place
Difficulty Level: Low.
Special Emphasis or Benefits: Easy lymphatic flow and immune system booster.

General Description: With Easy Bouncing, you merely stand on the rebounder and push down with your core torso muscles and a bit with your lower legs, generating an up-and-down motion. Your feet, your legs, your torso, and your arms stay pretty much in the same position as your entire body descends into the mat a few inches down and then comes back up to where you started. One way to initiate this bounce is to stand on the rebounder and then, as you exhale, emphasize the contraction of your abdominals while pushing down with them through your legs. Note that your feet—at least your toes—are staying on the mat the whole time, with perhaps your heels lifting off just one or two inches.

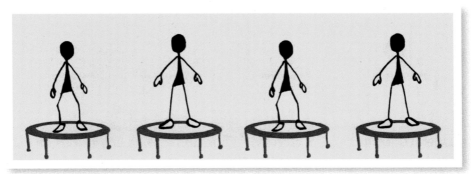

Comments: This is about the simplest Bounce Type possible. Note that the feet do sink into the mat here, so there is an actual up-and-down pulsing motion and vertical displacement of the body. Generally, the arms will not move very much, but they may be needed for balance. This is an excellent movement to perform while also practicing Breathwork Bouncing.

Variation # 1: Try putting your feet closer together, even right next to each other, or separating them as far as they will go while remaining on the mat.

Variation # 2: Place your feet in a "V" configuration, with heels together and toes separated, or with toes together and heels separated. You can also try the various positions of ballet (e.g., first position, second position) while Pulsing in Place.

Variation # 3: Loosely hold a light weight in each hand as you're Pulsing in Place and see what the extra weight feels like added to your body in the up-and-down motions.

Easy Bouncing # 2: Alternate Feet Shuffle
Difficulty Level: Low to medium (including variations).
Special Emphasis or Benefits: Easy immune system boost; some aerobic effect.

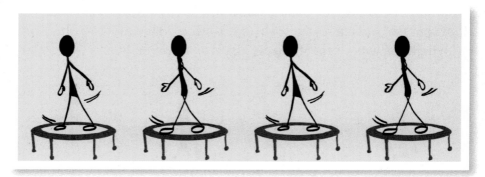

General Description: Stand on the rebounder, feet a bit apart, arms hanging at your sides. Then move one foot forward on a straight line as you move your other foot backward. You will sink into the mat when your feet are farthest apart, and then come up again as they are passing each other. You can let your arms swing back and forth or not—whatever feels best to you.

Comments: This movement is reminiscent of taking a stroll in a park. This is another excellent movement to do while practicing Breathwork Bouncing.

Variation # 1: Consciously swing your arms with your feet, moving your right arm forward as your right foot goes forward, and your left arm backward as your left foot goes backward, and vice versa.

Variation # 2: This time, swing your arms in the opposite direction—that is, as your right foot goes forward your left arm goes forward, and so on. Note that by moving opposite arms and legs forward and backward, you're performing a cross-crawl motion, which is said to help with left brain/right brain integration.

Variation # 3: Start with your feet horizontally closer together (up to right next to each other) or spread farther apart (farther than shoulder width apart).

Variation # 4: Experiment with how far you vertically displace your feet (e.g., do they barely change places with respect to which one is farther forward, or is there a substantial gap by the time one foot has moved all the way forward and the other has moved all the way backward?). You can also experiment with how far you swing your arms backward and forward.

Easy Bouncing # 3: Legs and Feet Twist
Difficulty Level: Medium.
Special Emphasis or Benefits: Engages core muscles, arms, and shoulders.

General Description: Stand on the rebounder, feet a bit apart, arms hanging at your sides. Then simply twist your legs and feet in one direction as you allow your arms and torso to naturally swing in the other. Your feet do not leave the mat, but you will naturally sink into the mat as you end the twist in each direction.

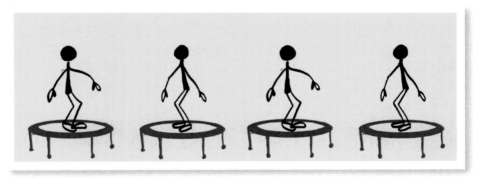

Comments: This is an easy and powerful movement that engages your body in a beneficial cross-crawl motion. In addition to focusing on your legs and feet to generate the twist, you can also focus on your core torso muscles and generate the twist mainly from there (that is, try initiating the movement from your core). Let your arms swing freely as your body moves.

Variation # 1: Start with your feet horizontally closer together (up to right next to each other) or spread farther apart (farther than shoulder width apart).

Variation # 2: (If you're susceptible to cartilage damage, especially medial meniscus damage, don't try this variation.) With your feet close together (as in Variation # 1), try pressing your knees and thighs together as you twist. Please note that, although they are not always specifically pointed out, there are many Bounce Types throughout this chapter that, if you hold your knees and thighs together as you bounce, will help you experience that movement in a surprisingly different and often beneficial way.

Variation # 3: Focus on twisting from your core with gusto—really feel your abdominals and core muscles as the part of you that generates the twist. But make sure you're fully aligned and strong throughout your body before you put too much energy into this. (Always let pain be your guide. If you start to feel like you're doing too much, then slow down or stop what you're doing completely and transition into some other motion.)

Variation # 4: Experiment with how far you swing your arms. Does it feel different if you hold them close versus giving them an extra big swing in each direction? How about if you lift your arms vertically up and down or even alternate them as they swing up and down? See how that changes the motion of your body and affects your core muscles.

B. Breathwork Bouncing

Breathwork Bouncing lies close to the true heart of rebounding as a health and wellness practice. Breath is intimately tied to physical, psychological, and even spiritual well-being. And while breathing is the simplest thing in the world—we all do it automatically and autonomically, roughly 23,000 times a day on average[16]—many people have breathing patterns that are dysfunctional or at least far less than optimal. If you can get a better handle on breathing while you're bouncing, it's likely that some of that better breathing will start showing up in other parts of your life: in play, under stress or even duress, and perhaps even when you're just sitting down.

The bottom line for breathwork is for you to be—or become—aware of your breathing, relax your neck and shoulders, and allow your abdominals, stomach, and entire pelvic region to relax as well. You can tuck your

---

16   See http://www.heraldtribune.com/article/20100112/ARTICLE/1121008.

pelvis under a tad[17] and make sure you're tall, long, and aligned, but forget about being "fat"; forget about having a "waist"; forget about everything but allowing as much air as possible to regularly come in and out of your central body cavity. When you fully breathe in through your nose, when your diaphragm expands fully, you will have more of a "belly" than usual, and that's great! You're the big-bellied Buddha, laughing at how wonderful it is to breathe fully! Breath is life: let as much of it come into and through you as possible.

Please note that most of the examples of Breathwork Bouncing provided here can be done—and in fact must be done—along with other Bounce Types. That is, you add or layer on a component of Breathwork Bouncing to some other Bounce Type that you're doing. The three Bounce Type examples (plus variations) considered for the Breathwork Bouncing category are:

1. Awareness Breathing
2. Patterned Breathing
3. Work-It-Through Breathing

Breathwork Bouncing # 1: Awareness Breathing
Difficulty Level: Low to high.
Special Emphasis or Benefits: Body and mind awareness; facilitates healing.

General Description: At any point in any rebounding session, regardless of the Bounce Type that you're engaged in, you can become fully aware of your breathing (if you aren't already). Just watch your breath—gently place your attention on your breath—and ask yourself some questions:

---

17 For general instruction on standing, sitting, walking, driving, sleeping, and breathing well throughout all of these activities, the work of Esther Gokhale and the Gokhale Method is highly recommended; see http://egwellness.com. One of Esther's important teachings is that in most situations, better posture and breathing require an anteverted pelvis, that is, one where you're sticking out a little in a "duck butt" position, which is the **opposite** of tucking your pelvis. So you'll want to experiment with breath and comfort, and find some position that is neither too tucked nor too sticking out, depending on the kind of bouncing you are doing.

- Does my breath come regularly and easily?
- Is it full?
- Am I inhaling completely?
- Exhaling completely?
- Is my breath stuck anywhere in my body?
- If there is any pain or soreness or "stuck" feeling anywhere in my body, and does my breath go to that place or go around that place?
- Does anything change if I imagine or visualize my breath going into that place so it can be worked with or healed?

Comments: It's easier to watch your breath with the simpler Bounce Types, such as those in the Easy Bouncing or Going-with-the-Flow categories (we'll get to the latter pretty soon), but you truly can learn to just watch your breath at any point while bouncing. Tied in to watching your breath is noticing where your body is tight. Typical places for holding and constriction include the neck, shoulders, abdominal region, and the whole pelvic region. Awareness Breathing does not call for you to make any changes to what you're doing in real time. Instead, the notion here is that awareness itself is helpful, healthful, and happy-making.

Some people find watching their breath for a given period of time is pretty easy. For others, it's difficult to place consistent awareness on breathing for more than just a few breaths, which is why the difficulty level for Awareness Breathing ranges from low to high. As you master Awareness Breathing, you may want to experiment more with Patterned Breathing, which is the next step in Breathwork Bouncing.

Variation # 1: Place a clock where you can easily see it and decide that you're going to remain aware of your breathing for a certain minimum amount of time—say two minutes. Practice until you do not lose awareness of your breath during that minimum period. Then increase the duration until you reach five to 10 minutes of awareness, or even longer. And if it sounds to you like this would be easy and kind of boring...well...give it a try anyway. You might find it isn't so easy, or that you will experience or learn some very interesting things if you just give it a go.

Variation # 2: Again using a clock, spend the first two to three minutes of each rebounding session, as well as the last two to three minutes, practicing Awareness Breathing. In this way—focusing on breath both at the start and at the finish—you can build the habit of regularly returning to awareness of your breathing while bouncing.

Breathwork Bouncing # 2: Patterned Breathing
Difficulty Level: Medium to high.
Special Emphasis or Benefits: Body and mind awareness; facilitates healing.

General Description: Unlike Awareness Breathing, which only requires watching and then placing attention on the breath, Patterned Breathing involves not only watching, but purposefully timing your inhales and exhales. Fortunately, rebounding provides us with a kind of built-in metronome. Every time your feet hit the mat, you can count it as a single beat, which makes it easy to "time" Bounce Types when you want to do so.

As with the other Breathwork Bounces, Patterned Breathing can be done with many different Bounce Types, including Pulsing in Place, Just Bouncin', Jumping Jacks, any of the various Twists, Handheld Weights Bouncing, and so on. While there are many different Breathwork patterns that can be used, we recommend trying the following patterns first as you layer them on top of some of the Bounce Types mentioned above:

- **Two-Step:** Switch between inhaling and exhaling on every bounce cycle; that is, every time your feet hit the mat, change from inhale to exhale. This rapid pattern, somewhat reminiscent of the yogic "breath of fire," can become very intense and difficult to hold for very long.
- **Two-Count:** Inhale to a count of two (your feet hitting the mat twice), then exhale for a count of two.
- **Three-Count:** Inhale for a count of three, then exhale for a count of three.
- **Four-Count, Five-Count, etc.:** Inhale for the number of counts you determine, then exhale for the same number of counts

- **Increase Then Decrease Count:** Starting with a two-count, inhale and then exhale to successively larger numbers of counts, stopping when you find you have reached your limit, and then count back down until you reach two again.

Comments: Breathe in and out completely as you do with any Patterned Breathing. If you're breathing in and out to too long a count, you won't be able to perform full inhales or exhales, which is a good indication that you need to cut back. If you can get up to a five-count, that's pretty darn good.

Variation # 1: Do a Two-Step Patterned Breathing count to any of the Jumping Jacks, exhaling each time your arms come down and your legs come together. Now reverse this—exhale each time your arms go up and your legs separate—and see which way feels easier and more natural. But challenge yourself to do it the other way as well.

Variation # 2: Do a Two-Step Patterned Breathing count while using hand weights to do an Overhead Press. Here, exhale each time your arms go above your head and inhale as they come down. It is generally easier and more natural when using hand weights to exhale as your arms move up and away from (or out from) your torso.

Note: There are many, many other breathwork patterns you can explore. For example, Molly Hale of Ability Production (see http://abilityproduction.org) taught Jordan a very potent healing breathwork pattern. You breathe in for four full counts, then hold in for seven full counts, then exhale for eight full counts. This can be pretty intense, so you want to work your way into it slowly, perhaps first practicing it while you're sitting down or walking, and only then move it over to your bouncer with some Easy Bouncing.

Breathwork Bouncing # 3: Work-It-Through Breathing
Difficulty Level: Very individual, from low to very high.
Special Emphasis or Benefits: Facilitates healing and a sense of well-being.

General Description: While you are doing a set of any Bounce Type, you may find or become aware of a part of your body—whether muscle, connective tissue, an organ, or a body system—that feels restricted, constricted, "stuck," or painful or is otherwise just "not quite right," or NQR. Place your attention on that spot or body system and consciously breathe in and through that spot. Relaxing your neck, shoulders, pelvis, and abdomen, allow as much breath in and through all of you as possible. Imagine your full breath flushing through and taking away the pain or NQRness, which is then released into the earth each time you hit the bottom of your descent, and then call for healing energy from the heavens each time you rise to the top of your trajectory.

If breath alone does not completely diminish the pain or NQR feeling, then allow your body to slightly move and rearrange itself so that the pain or NQR feeling isn't quite so strong. Then continue with deep, full breathing, and when all signs of the pain or NQR feeling are gone, return to your original position and see if the pain or NQR feeling is now gone from this position as well. You can go back and forth between the original position and similar but different positions, consciously breathing through and letting go of the pain, as many times as you need to.

Once the pain or NQRness is mostly or completely gone, go ahead and see whether any of the pain or NQR feeling remains in your body by allowing your body to rearrange itself and go where it wants to go, including changing the Bounce Type that you're doing. The pain or NQR feeling may have traveled down to your knees, or up to your shoulders, or may have gone somewhere else in your body. If it has traveled, then keep "working it through" using your breath and slight changes in your body position.

Comments: Breath, pleasure, balance, and wellness are intimately related. By bringing yourself to a place where the air is flowing freely through your body, with your predominant feeling being a sense of clear and balanced presence and even pleasure, you give your body a kind of energetic template that can keep you healthy, balanced, and strong. If you end up often feeling terrific while you're bouncing, it's no doubt in part because you're breathing better and better, and you will likely find yourself breathing better than you used to when you're not bouncing as well.

This description of Work-It-Through Breathing may be a bit long-winded...but that's exactly the point. As you bring deep, full breathing—a long wind—in and through your body, and as you work with the edges of "stuckness," NQRness, and pain, including tracking down and releasing dysfunctional patterns wherever they may "travel" to as you do this work, you can deeply energize yourself and even heal long-standing problems and patterns. Each one of us will do Work-It-Through Breathing very differently, so take a deep breath and give yourself plenty of room to experiment with what works best.

C. Bodywork Bouncing

Bodywork Bouncing includes any type of self-administered hands-on bodywork that can be done during a rebounding session. It turns out that by applying your own hands, fingers, and fists to parts of your body while you're bouncing, you can give yourself an invigorating experience that will at least feel good and at best lead to healing or rehabilitation. Bodywork Bouncing can also be used hand in hand (or, perhaps, hand and nose) with Breathwork Bouncing, as previously described.

Given the many schools and types of self-massage, Touch for Health, Reiki, acupressure, and so on, it's no surprise that self-administered touch during a rebounding session might have positive effects. This can be an essential part of your bouncing repertoire, using Bodywork Bouncing movements to warm up and cool down as well as throughout your bouncing sessions.

This type of therapeutic approach helps elevate a regular workout to something that is not just sustainable but truly healing. Bodywork Bouncing movements can be especially useful for fibromyalgia or for injury recovery, but can also be used for the moderate muscle soreness that arises in everyday life. Go ahead and experiment and see if you can come up with any new types of Bodywork Bouncing that meet your needs and engage your enthusiasm and creativity.

The four Bounce Type examples (plus variations) for Bodywork Bouncing are:

1. Holding
2. Pressing
3. Tapping
4. Slapping

Bodywork Bouncing # 1: Holding

Difficulty Level: Low.

Special Emphasis or Benefits: Facilitates greater body awareness; inherent self-healing potential is often said to be found in the hands.

General Description: While Pulsing in Place (covered above), Just Bouncin' (covered below in the next section), or doing just about any other simple bounce that doesn't involve your arms or a great deal of your legs or torso, you can put your hands on or over your heart (image A), your navel (image B), behind your head (image C), or your lower back or hips (image D).

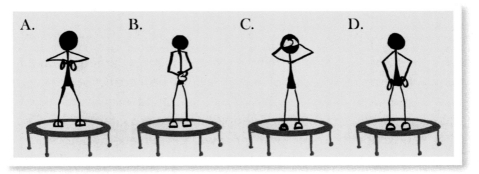

Comments: Here you simply hold the body part in question or place your hands over it. It can be helpful to imagine energy coming into your hands and warming or strengthening the area you're holding. If you also place attention on your breathing, you may experience not only greater body awareness but an awareness of the healing of dysfunctional or blocked physical or energetic patterns.

You can hold or put your hands over any part of your body, but four par-ticularly desirable areas to start with are:

- The lower back (where you can place your palms on your hips and your thumbs toward the small of your back, as in image D above)
- Your navel area (said to be the seat of power and will in many spiritual traditions)
- Your heart (whose importance goes without saying)
- Behind the head (where you can also press your thumbs into chron-ically tight muscles on the side of your neck)

As an experiment, start with some ordinary Pulsing in Place or Just Bouncin' (which we'll get to shortly), and then try putting your hands behind your head while continuing with the movement you've chosen. Feel how your body changes as you do this. From your muscles and bones to your soft tissue and fascia, the simple act of lifting your hands up behind your head will change how you use nearly all of your body in at least a few small ways. If you breathe deeply into and through this new position—breathing in and out fully through several cycles while holding your hands in this way—you may learn a great deal about your body and how it works. You may also have the opportunity to let go of some of the "stuck" or dysfunctional energy, patterns, and even physical structures that cause you pain or block you from optimal embodiment.

There is a great worldwide tradition of healing that is brought about and catalyzed through touch, including self-touch. The mere act of placing your hands on whatever part you choose may help bring energy and healing to that part or body system. Some people like to vigorously rub the palms of their hands together to generate more warmth and energy before placing their hands on their body. Of course, there are a wide variety of warming and healing herbal and medicinal rubs that can also be used (but be careful about your eyes and other orifices if you go that route).

Note that there's not all that much difference between Holding and the next Bounce Type, Pressing, and you may find yourself crossing over from one to the other. For example, if you press your thumbs into those muscles on the side of your neck as you're bouncing, and use the self-energizing property of bouncing on a rebounder to regularly but nearly effortlessly massage the area in question, you may get a wonderful sense of relief and tension reduction. Always use pain as your guide, of course, but you may find that many parts of your body enjoy being held or pressed for 15 or 20 seconds at a time or even longer. Aim for (a) staying symmetrical and (b) practicing good full breathing, while (c) making sure your overall posture and form are good.

Variations: Try Holding behind your head while pressing your knees together as you bounce up and down (if you can do this pain free). This really opens up the lower back, and can give you a profound perspective on how you normally "hold" your body!

Bodywork Bouncing # 2: Pressing
Difficulty Level: Medium.
Special Emphasis or Benefits: Facilitates greater body awareness; reha-bilitation and healing potential.

General Description: This is similar to Holding. Here, however, instead of just putting your hands onto or over a body part, you actually press into a part of your body that can benefit from the pressure delivered by a firm self-massage. When you use your fists, it becomes easy to stimulate the body part being pressed by taking advantage of the natural up-and-down rhythms mechanically generated by your rebounder. Or you can use your thumbs, depending on which part of yourself you're working on.

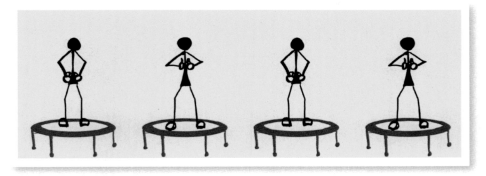

Comments: In the images above, the figure's fists start out pressing into their hips, and then they move up to the mid-back. You can keep your fists in any one place as long as you like, or move them up and down every several bounces as suggested in these images. When doing this kind of work, it's important to stay aware of your breath and keep your neck, shoulders, pelvis, and abdomen relaxed. As for how hard to press, this depends on what you're comfortable with and what works for you. Some people have much higher tolerance for pressure (and pain) than others, and it's important to remember to listen to your body on what feels right. As always, do what feels good, and pay careful attention to how your body feels when you're done with this Bounce Type.

Variation # 1: As suggested in the description of Holding, try Pressing into the sides of your neck with your thumbs.

Variation # 2: Try Pressing into your lower back, with your knees and thighs held some or all of the way together.

Bodywork Bouncing # 3: Tapping
Difficulty Level: Medium.
Special Emphasis or Benefits: Energizes and opens the breath and the body.

General Description: As you do a simple bounce—e.g., Pulsing in Place or Just Bouncin' (see below)—use your fingertips to lightly tap on your torso in different places. In the images below, the tapping moves from down near the navel to the hips and thighs, next to the shoulders, and then to the heart. You can tap all over the body, even the top of your head, to awaken all the energy stored up there!

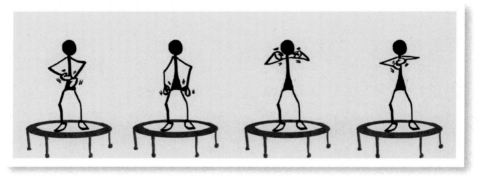

Comments: When you tap on your body with your fingertips, you encourage full breathing and body awareness. Not only does energy seem to "move through" and invigorate the body, but it becomes easier to observe how you're breathing and then to consciously participate in your breathing patterns. Tap lightly but firmly, moving the tapping up and down your torso, making sure that you keep your neck and shoulders, as well as your pelvis and abdomen, as relaxed as you can.

Variation # 1: There is an entire world of "energy psychology" therapeutic techniques, such as "Thought Field Therapy" and "Emotional Freedom Technique" (EFT), based on using fingertips to gently tap on acupuncture meridian points. While the founder of EFT, Gary Craig, passed away some time ago, his website is still going strong and offers complete free instructions on how to tap.[18] By now, there are many controlled studies showing that tapping is effective for a wide variety of maladies, from headaches to phobias.[19]

As you bounce, simply tap right at about your hip bones (or, really, anywhere else on your body) with what have been called the "karate chop points" on the sides of your hands. Make firm but loving contact with your body as you hold your hands as tightly or loosely as you like. (You may find a certain range of tension that feels best, e.g., where your hands begin to curl into a tight-knit form but still remain fairly loose and flexible.) By doing this kind of tapping, it is said that you may be able to counter or neutralize any experience you may be having of "psychological reversal" (where you've been feeling down or depressed, as if you were "mis-wired" and unable to get grounded and get on the right track). For those so inclined, try adding in an affirmation, visualization, chant, intention, or prayer. You never know what's going to spring loose the magic...

Variation # 2: Tap on other parts of the body than the ones described above. Try places on your back, on your sides, and wherever else you're drawn to and can safely reach while you're bouncing. Some areas, like the eyes, obviously are off limits or should only be tapped very, very lightly. Go gently on your kidneys as well.

Variation # 3: Instead of tapping by volitionally moving your hands and fingers (or the side of your hand in the case of the karate chop points) to a spot on the body, try holding your hands or fingers steady *and bounce yourself into them.* In other words, on the upward part of each up-and-down cycle, if you hold your hands and fingers steady, parts of your body will naturally come into contact with them. This is a delightful and very different way of making contact with yourself.

Notes: The simple mechanical devices known as Bongers are also great for doing this kind of tapping work as well as the Slapping described below. With flexible plastic or metal handles and rubber or plastic balls at the end, they can be used in many stimulating, therapeutic, and pleasurable ways.

18   See http://www.emofree.com/eft-tutorial/tapping-basics/how-to-do-eft.html.
19   See, e.g., http://articles.mercola.com/sites/articles/archive/2013/12/26/emotional -freedom-technique.aspx.

Bodywork Bouncing # 4: Slapping
Difficulty Level: Medium.
Special Emphasis or Benefits: Wakes up the body's energy!

General Description: Much like Tapping, Slapping wakes up the body's energies—stimulating it directly to let it know it's alive. The main difference is that instead of just using your fingertips, you use the palms of your hands and stimulate your body vigorously by literally slapping parts of yourself (safe parts, and only with an appropriate amount of force). It is usually done with Pulsing in Place, Just Bouncin', or any simple bounce that does not require twisting of the torso or use of the arms and hands to do other things.

In the images below, we show you various types of Slapping: A is Slapping your thighs, B is Slapping your glutes, C is Slapping your abdomen, and D is Slapping your legs while your arms swing back and forth. You can even (moderately!) slap your neck and your face to wake them up as well. Listen to what your body is asking for, and then go for it.

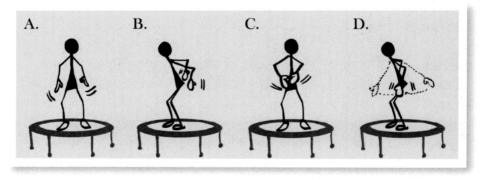

Comments: Slapping can sound a little odd to the uninitiated, and can look even odder to those who sees you doing it. But don't worry about other people; as we suggested elsewhere, many people prefer to do their bouncing—especially things like Tapping and Slapping—alone. The question is what works, feels good, and is beneficial for you.

Slapping can be surprisingly invigorating and is certainly well worth trying. It doesn't have to be the kind of slap where you redden your skin or leave any marks. We suggest trying out different degrees of force to see what feels good. Even light Slapping can move a lot of energy and awareness through your body. Be open and see what is useful for you.

Variation # 1: Just as you can Tap up and down the body, as described earlier, you can also Slap up and down the body, although you may want to Slap with less force on your torso and head than you would on naturally "padded" areas like the glutes.

‖ *D. Flow Bouncing*

The category of Flow Bouncing—short for "Going with the Flow" Bouncing—includes bounces that you can always turn to when you find yourself in or approaching a "flow" state in the middle of a rebounding session. "Flow," as the term's originator Professor Mihaly Csikszentmihalyi puts it, is a "sense of effortless action [people] feel in moments that stand out as the best in their lives. Athletes refer to it as being in the zone, religious mystics as being in ecstasy, artists and musicians as aesthetic rapture."[20]

Such Flow Bouncing experiences can constitute an increasing portion of your Basic Bounces over time, as they tend to naturally and easily arise and build the kind of effortless pleasurable momentum that leads to sustained periods of "timeless" bouncing.

To keep things interesting, remember that you can always significantly alter any one of these Bounce Types by making a slight change in the positions of your hands, your shoulders, your arms, your feet, and so on. (And on top of that, you can always layer on a little bit of intentional Breathwork, as described in chapter 7's discussion of Layering and Gearing.)

Five examples of Flow Bouncing are:
1. Just Bouncin'
2. Jumping Jacks
3. The Twist
4. Arm Circles
5. Free-Flow Feel Good

---

20 *Finding Flow* by Mihaly Csikszentmihalyi (1997), p. 29.
    See also https://en.wikipedia.org/wiki/Mihaly_Csikszentmihalyi.

Flow Bouncing # 1: Just Bouncin'
Difficulty Level: Low.
Special Emphasis or Benefits: Perfect for when you just...want...to bounce.

General Description: Sometimes when you're rebounding you don't want to think too hard, work too hard, or pay too much attention to anything in particular. Instead, you just want to be bouncing. Just Bouncin' is bound to be just the right answer for these times. Using mainly your core torso muscles along with your lower legs (and, of course, feet), you push down to push off. As you consistently push off—even just a little bit—you'll develop a nice, easy, natural rhythm that makes you feel not only pretty good, but like you really wouldn't want to be doing anything else anyway.

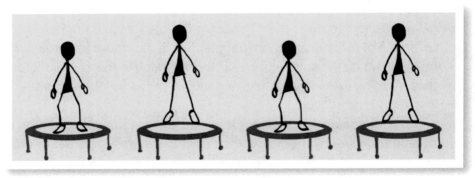

Comments: Just Bouncin' makes for smooth transitions, especially when you're in the middle of a rebounding session. If you're not sure what you want to do next, you can always just start Just Bouncin'.

Variation # 1: Do some Breathwork Bouncing as you are Just Bouncin'.

Variation # 2: You can hold light hand weights as you are Just Bouncin', which will help you tone/build muscle and burn more calories.

Variation # 3: With a little bit more lower-leg push-off, you're halfway to High Bouncing; that is, you're Just Bouncin' higher.

Flow Bouncing # 2: Jumping Jacks
Difficulty Level: Low to medium.
Special Emphasis or Benefits: Easy, simple, natural, and uses the whole body.

General Description: This is similar to the well-known callisthenic move-ment that we've all done at some point in our lives, except (of course) that you're bouncing as you do it. Simply move your arms apart and overhead as you spread your legs, then bring your hands and arms back overhead as your legs come back together.

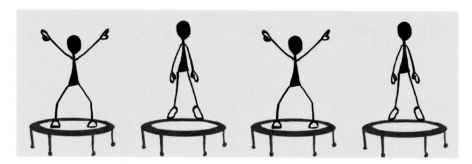

Comments: In a traditional callisthenic jumping jack on a hard surface, the hands meet overhead. Some of the variations below have the hands meeting overhead in different ways, but for a standard execution of Jump-ing Jacks, you only need to raise your arms most of the way above your head. In other words, as part of the Flow Bouncing category of Bounce Types—bounces that you can come back to over and over again—simple Jumping Jacks as shown above are indeed simple, easy, and quite natural on a rebounder.

Variation # 1: If, however, you want to stay closer to the traditional callis-thenic, and you can do it with no strain, then have your hands meet gently overhead, and your shoulders and back will get an especially nice workout.

Variation # 2: In addition to bringing your hands to meet each other as you do with basic Jumping Jacks, there are variations that change the feel and effect of the movement, depending on exactly how your hands meet each other. For example, you can clap your hands as they reach their apex overhead. And as for the clapping, you can clap with your hands flat, or you can clap by nestling four of your fingers into the thumb of one hand, and then on the next bounce cycle switch which hand is the "nestler" and which is the "nestlee." Switching back and forth between hands as you clap brings a rewarding and challenging rhythm to Jumping Jacks.

Variation # 3: Turning or rotating your hands and wrists 90 degrees or more in either direction will give you a nice variation that emphasizes shoulder and arm work and really helps stretch out both your arms as well. Note, though, that you won't be able to clap normally once you've fully rotated your arms and shoulders one way or the other.

Variation # 4: Jumping Jacks are so much fun because there are so many different ways to do them while you're bouncing. In another variation, your hands and arms cross over each other, first left arm in front of right, then right arm in front of left. This not only brings more of a neurological challenge, but is fun to do.

Variation # 5: Another thing you can do differently with your hands during Jumping Jacks is *let your hands completely relax*. They will seem to flutter or flop as you move your arms, especially at the top of the bounce. Allow any tension in your wrists or fingers to let go, and let them move however they seem to want to. It may look a little goofy to an outsider,[21] but this can be a lot of fun, and you can discharge a lot of tightness from your hands, wrists, and arms in this way.

Variation # 6: You can also try *switching the timing of your arms and legs*. Normally, your arms and hands go up as your feet and legs spread apart. Here, the timing is switched, with the feet coming together as the arms and hands reach their highest point, and the feet spreading out as the arms come down. While this may sound easy, it can prove pretty challenging at first, as the way you've done jumping jacks your whole life will attempt to reassert itself.

---

21   We've said it before, but we want to say it again: Rebounding around others, especially if they don't bounce themselves and aren't used to what the Bounce entails, can be a bit challenging. Ultimately, you're bouncing for you, and you shouldn't let the thoughts or reactions of others dissuade you from choosing to take care of yourself.

Variation # 7: Variations can also include changes in the feet and legs. For example, try spreading your feet open in a kind of V, your toes pointing at roughly 10 o'clock and 2 o'clock, and then on the next bounce cycle close them back in to parallel and pointing forward (or you can even turn your toes slightly inward and begin to create a kind of reverse V shape). This is a great way to open up your hip flexors and stretch all the ligaments and muscles on the sides of your legs.

Variation # 8: As a last and final variation, you can get really crazy. Instead of moving your arms only up and down along your sides, you can swing them down in front of your body. Begin as you would with a regular Jumping Jack. When your hands are at the highest point, bring both your arms down in front of you. Then swing them back up the same way they just came down, and at the highest point again bring your arms back down along your sides. Moving your arms back and forth between the two positions like this while you're otherwise doing your Jumping Jacks is a great way to rotate your shoulders and open up the upper back. Get extra fancy by placing your legs wide apart or moving your feet in and out as described above at the same time.

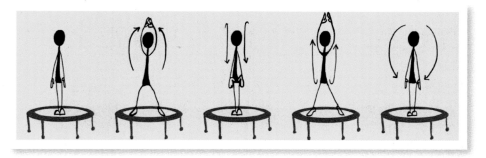

Flow Bouncing # 3: The Twist
Difficulty Level: Low to medium.
Special Emphasis or Benefits: Intensely engages core torso muscles.

General Description: Stand on your rebounder, bend your knees slightly, and rotationally twist your arms and torso in one direction while your hips and legs begin to move in the opposite direction. Think: corkscrew.

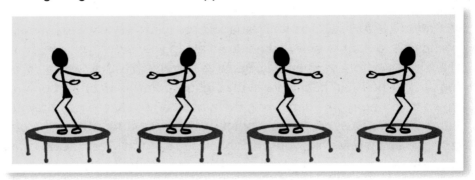

Comments: Right up there with Jumping Jacks and Just Bouncin', there may be no more natural, beneficial, and enjoyable Bounce Type than the Twist. It's very easy to start twisting on a rebounder, yet the Twist can also challenge you both structurally and aerobically. Not surprisingly, there are many ways to do the Twist.

Variation # 1: Move your arms back and forth above your body as you Twist. This is the "Windshield Wiper Twist," and it will give you some nice shoulder and arm movement.

Variation # 2: "Twist Over Head" is similar to the 50's dance known as "The Monkey." You bring your hands up and over your head, either straight or in an arcing motion. This is a lot of fun, especially with the right music, and it gives the shoulders and mid to upper back an excellent workout.

Variation # 3: In "Low Back Twist," you bend your knees deeper while you're twisting, and your arms move back and forth in front of you instead of going all the way behind you. You can get a really thorough lower back stretch from this as well as working your quadriceps, depending on how low you go with your knees. (But don't go too low! Use pain as your guide.) This can give you a lot of very good, rewarding work.

Flow Bouncing # 4: Arm Circles
Difficulty Level: Low to medium.
Special Emphasis or Benefits: Engages shoulders, upper back, neck, and arms.

General Description: Stand on your rebounder, start pulsing or bouncing with a little bit of vertical lift, stretch out your arms and hands, and then start making circles with your hands and arms, either forward (Illustration A) or backward (Illustration B).

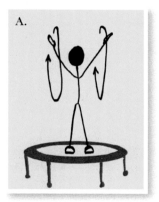
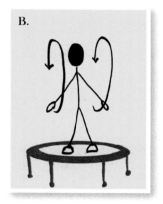

Comments: It's important to start with small arm circles, and then you can make them wider and wider over time, bringing in more of your shoulders and back. Make sure to really *feel* into just how big a circle you can make—but if you feel any real pain, then back off. It's also important to change directions; that is, go both forward and backward with your arms. If you do 50 Arm Circles frontward, then do 50 Arm Circles backward.

Variation # 1: Later on, after practicing Arm Circles without weights, try adding in light handheld weights—no more than one or two pounds at first.

No Need to Shoulder That Pain and
Stay All Torn Up Any Longer
Once upon a time I (Jordan) tore my rotator cuff after getting tangled up in some garden weeds. I heard/felt something tear, and after being examined, was told that it was my rotator cuff. I went for many physical therapy

sessions, but they weren't helping that much. So I stopped going to physical therapy, thinking it would take months and months to fully heal.

Fortunately, I was then inspired to try progressively larger and larger arm circles—100 in each direction, every day. Within just a few weeks of bouncing like this, nearly all of the pain and immobility associated with my torn rotator cuff went away. And while this may be just an anecdotal account, I wouldn't hesitate to recommend arm circles in both directions for anyone suffering from this condition or other kinds of shoulder immobility.

Flow Bouncing # 5: Free-Flow Feel Good
Difficulty Level: Low.
Special Emphasis or Benefits: Invites the mind and body to completely relax.

General Description: While rebounding, you will sometimes just want to do what feels spontaneously good and natural, even and especially if it doesn't fit into any other Bounce Type. If this comes up, then just go with it (pretty much always). The natural, spontaneous, organic movements that arise within you are thoroughly enjoyable, and can relax you and open you up in ways that can lead to deep energizing and healing. Of course, you want to maintain some level of observing yourself and take care not to go too wild or move your neck too freely and crazily.

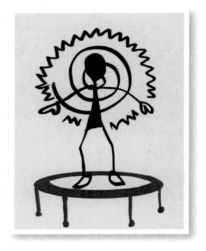

Comments: If at any time you happen to find yourself having super fun while bouncing—let's say things are flowing freely, and you're feeling really good—then try not to even think of questioning what you're doing or how good it feels. After all, this is a large part of why you got on a rebounder in the first place! A fun, easy way to fitness!

Type 2: Expanded Bounces—Intermediate and Accessory-Based Bounces

A. Bouncing with Handheld Weights, Gloves, and Other Accessories

Many people—female, male, and nonbinary—ask whether rebounding will keep their upper body in shape, especially their arm and chest muscles. Our experience is that the very mechanics of rebounding adds core muscle to the torso and otherwise produce excellent muscle tone throughout the entire body.[22] (Consider that you use both legs in every bounce—except if you're bouncing one-legged—and you can easily see why legs that bounce tend to be toned and strong.) Moreover, if strength is seen in the context of flexibility and the ability to powerfully but safely navigate your body through the challenges of everyday life, then rebounding will certainly improve overall strength.

To target specific muscle groups, you can add handheld weights of various types to your bouncing routine to gain extra strength and benefit from all of the things that weight-bearing exercise does for your overall health and body. Additionally, just as you would do workouts in the gym that focus on specific muscle groups, you can target your rebounding exercise to build strength and tone in more isolated areas. The added bonus, however, is that not only are you working that isolated muscle group, as in a bicep curl for example, but the whole rest of your body is involved as well, sub-stantially increasing the effectiveness of your workout.

The upshot is that you can indeed give yourself an intense upper-body workout focused on the chest, arms, shoulders, and back. But don't use anything like the same kind of weight you'd normally use at the gym! The addition of gravity acting upon the weight as you bounce up and down—especially when you reverse directions—increases the weight's perceived heaviness quite a bit. (Think of your elbow and shoulder as being fulcrums, with any handheld weight pressing down with quite a bit of leverage as you reach the end of your range of motion and reverse directions.)

---

22 Chapter 8's "Jordan's Journal" presents some new ideas and includes a detailed overall discussion on why rebounding seems to be so good at toning and building muscle.

Start light—and we mean really light—with one- or two-pound weights. (Regular dumbbells are easiest to get ahold of, but other options include D-shaped dumbbells, one- or at most two-pound weighted gloves[23] that strap on with Velcro, and women's Shake Weights, as discussed earlier.) This may seem like a very small amount of weight at first, especially if you're a seasoned weight lifter or have always been athletic, strong, and healthy, but the burn that comes from doing many repetitions at even such low weights will quickly convince you that it is, in fact, working. In the penultimate chapter of this book, Jordan will have more to say about his latest thoughts as to why bouncing with handheld weights, progressively increasing the weight, seems to be so effective at toning and building muscle.

Remember, too, that compared to how you might regularly work with handheld weights, you'll be undertaking more repetitions and more sets than normal, thereby allowing your muscles to fatigue in a way that is dissimilar from what you may be used to in high-weight, low-repetition types of weight lifting (where the goal is often out-and-out muscle failure—you don't want any muscle failure while you're bouncing holding weights!).

Once you feel that you've mastered a given weight, you can increase it a bit, perhaps moving from one to two pounds, or from two to three, or if you're really strong to begin with, from three to five pounds. If you have a set of graduated weights—one-pounders, two-pounders, three-pounders, etc.—you can also simply increase the poundage you're working with after a certain number of repetitions, or when you come back to that Bounce Type later in your workout.

Always remember to listen to your body. You're lifting on an unstable surface, which adds many variables that you don't experience when you're on solid ground. Pay attention to your joints and ligaments, and make sure you're strong enough to stabilize the weights that you have in your hand without hurting yourself. Keep your knees soft, your posture good, and your breath active and aware.

---

23   Velcro-enabled gloves appeal to some as a great way to add resistance while leaving your hands completely free, open, and relaxed. Generally, though, one-pound weighted gloves (such as the P90X brand) are best; anything heavier than that and the weighted gloves tend to be cumbersome, uncomfortable to wear, and difficult to put on.

You can also use equipment like kettlebells, resistance bands, and medicine balls while rebounding. For example, for working on the chest while bouncing, a "Pilates Ring"—a flexible rubber circle with handles on each side that can be compressed—works particularly well, and can be used in a wide variety of ways. The possibilities here are nearly endless, and you really can create a full-body, fully integrated, highly effective, resistance-based workout right in the comfort of your own home.

The five Bounce Type examples along with variations for the Handheld Weights Bouncing Category are:

1. Overhead Press
2. Arm Raise
3. Bicep Curls
4. Squats
5. Triceps

Handheld Weights Bouncing # 1: Overhead Press
Difficulty Level: Medium to high (depending on speed and number of reps).
Special Emphasis or Benefits: Shoulders, arms, chest, and back.

General Description: For the Overhead Press, pick up some light handheld weights (or strap on your weighted gloves), and with palms facing forward, raise your hands and the weights over your head as you bounce. Your feet (or just your heels) may leave the mat at the top of your extension and then come back into firm full contact with the mat again as you bring the weights down to roughly in line with the tops of your shoulders.

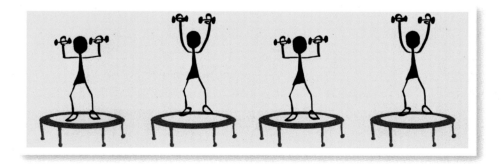

Comments: Make sure **you do not use weights that are too heavy**, especially at first. Pay attention to your breath and body (relax your neck, shoulders, pelvis, and abdominals, as always, and make sure that your breath is aware, alert, and active—and ideally mainly through the nose), and start out with 10 or 20 repetitions, eventually working up to dozens or even hundreds of repetitions, if you like. Done to music, with attention placed on the breath and good posture, this can be a very rewarding and intense movement.

Variation # 1: Shoulder Press with palms facing in. Keep your arms parallel to your body as above, but twist your hands in so that your palms are facing in toward your body as you hold the weights. Now extend your arms all the way up, just as before. Keep your palms facing in for the entire movement.

Variation # 2: The Arnold Press was invented by Arnold Schwarzenegger and is a great workout for both shoulders and upper chest. Begin with your arms bent, with your elbows tucked in by your sides and your hands (holding the weights) facing into your shoulders. Next, extend your arms up, and as you straighten your elbows, twist your hands so that your palms are now facing out and away from you. The top extension of this motion brings your arms straight in the air with your hands facing out in front of you. Next, bring your arms back down and twist your hands back so that you end up with your palms facing in toward your shoulders again.

Variation # 3: Single Arm Press. This is exactly the same as a regular shoulder press, but with one arm at a time. You can use a regular handheld weight or even a kettlebell. Try doing all of your repetitions on one side before switching to the other side. Or, as an alternative, alternate arms, switching back and forth.

Don't De-Feet Yourself When Starting Out With Handheld Weights

Don't think too much about or try to do too much with your feet when you are first practicing any movements using handheld weights.

Indeed, your feet can stay completely flat on the mat the whole time you're working with handheld weights or weight-related accessories of any type. Your center of gravity—in effect, all your weight, plus the weight associated with the handheld weights—will still be moving up and down and shifting direction even if you leave your feet completely flat the whole time.

When you're ready, you can begin by lifting your heels in sync with the rest of the movement you are doing, and then eventually perhaps go a step further and shoot for some vertical liftoff as you do any of these weights-enabled movements. Keep in mind, though, that if you do gain vertical liftoff, it will take a whole lot more energy and be much more intense.

Handheld Weights Bouncing # 2: Arm Raises
Difficulty Level: Medium to high (depending on speed and number of reps).
Special Emphasis or Benefits: Shoulders, forearms, wrists, chest, and back.

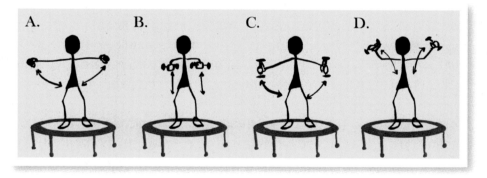

General Description: For the Arm Raise pictured in image A above, which is a general shoulder fly or lateral arm raise, pick up some light handheld weights (or just strap on your weighted gloves) and hold them with your palms facing inward toward the sides of your body. Keeping your elbows straight but not locked, raise your arms to the side as your feet (or just your heels) lift off the mat, with your feet coming into full contact with the mat again as you reach the top of your extension, which should have your arms just parallel to the floor, at shoulder level. Imagine making a "T" with your body. Then bring your arms down the exact same way, with the weights coming all the way down to pelvis level as your feet sink into and make full contact with the mat again.

Variation # 1: (Image B) Front Raise. Begin with your palms facing in and your arms straight down so that your elbows are almost touching your hips and your hands are resting on your thighs. Lift your arms straight up, keeping your elbows straight but not locked, and end so that your arms are parallel to the floor. Then return to the starting position.

Variation # 2: (Image C) Side Raise with palms facing forward. This is exactly like the first variation, but instead of having your palms facing in and down toward your body, your palms are facing out in front of you. Begin with your arms by your side and palms facing out. Raise your arms up straight, keeping your thumb on top the entire way. End the movement the same way you began.

Variation # 3: (Image D) Reverse Fly standing upright. This movement focuses a bit of loving attention on your rear deltoids and your trapezius, the back-most muscle that makes up your shoulder and the muscles that comprise your upper back. Begin with your palms facing down and your arms down in front of you, just like in Variation # 1. Keep a slight bend in your elbow and lift your arms so that they are parallel to the floor and out to the sides of your body. This means that your palms are now facing forward. Lower your arms and return to your starting position.

Comments: Again, make sure you read the comments in the introductory section on using handheld weights and be sure to use appropriate—that is, light—weights. Pay attention to your breath and body (relax the neck, shoulders, pelvis, and abdominals, as always), and start out with five or 10 repetitions, eventually working your way up to dozens, or a hundred, or more. These movements really work the shoulders intensely, as well as the forearms and wrists.

Place special attention on your neck and face, keeping them loose and relaxed as you perform these movements. This isn't always an easy thing to do: the Arm Raise group of exercises, if done for enough repetitions, is flat out very intense. (And, as described in chapter 8, it can produce muscle fatigue and get you close to muscle failure, which is what precedes muscle growth.) Nobody ever said that all of rebounding was going to be easy, but the results are definitely worth it!

Handheld Weights Bouncing # 3: Bicep Curls
Difficulty Level: Medium to high.
Special Emphasis or Benefits: Your biceps.

General Description: Grasp an appropriately light handheld weight in each hand. With each bounce, you'll be raising one or both of your arms, and then lowering that arm or arms on the next bounce (and if you're alternating and raising one arm at a time, as in Variation # 2, you'll be raising the other arm as your first arm goes down). Remember to keep your neck, shoulders, pelvis, and abdomen relaxed, and place some attention on your breathing.

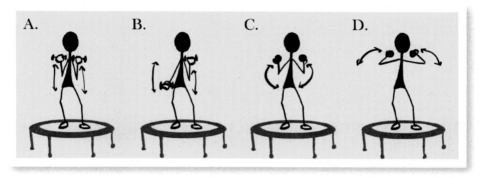

Variation # 1: (Image A) With both arms together, this variation is what you might think of as a regular bicep curl. Begin with your palms facing inward toward your thighs and arms straight along your sides. Flex your biceps and bend your elbows as you rotate your hands so that they are facing toward your shoulders at the top of the motion. Reverse the rotation to end where you began. You can do this up-and-down motion with each up-and-down of your bounce cycle, or you can vary the rhythm of it, holding up for two cycles, and then down for two cycles, etc.

Variation # 2: (Image B) Bicep Curl with alternating arms. This is exactly the same as the first variation, but here you're alternating your arms. While one arm is up at your shoulder, the other is down at your side, and vice versa.

Variation # 3: (Image C) Bicep Curl with shoulders rotated out. In this bicep curl, you begin with rotating your shoulders so that the insides of your arms face away from you. Lock them in this position as they will stay here throughout the entire movement. Your palms should be facing out as well. Flex your biceps and bring your palms up to your shoulders exactly like a regular bicep curl, but continue to keep your arms and your shoulders rotated out. Straighten out your arms and return to the starting position. Experience what this feels like and how different it is from the original bicep curl.

Variation # 4: (Image D) Bicep Curl with elbows up. Just as in the last image, bend your arms and raise them up, and rotate your shoulders so your upper arms are perpendicular to your body, making a T. Keep your shoulders and elbows in exactly the same place the whole time! Now straighten out your arms with your palms facing up to the ceiling or the sky, extending that T to its fullest capacity. Then bend your arms and return to the starting position, making sure you don't drop your elbows down along the way.

Handheld Weights Bouncing # 4: Squats
Difficulty Level: Medium to high.
Special Emphasis or Benefits: Legs and core.

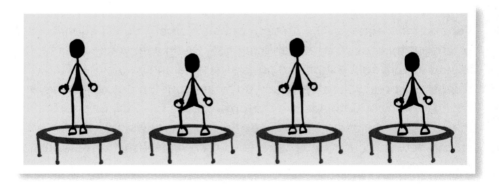

General Description: Squats are one of the most incorrectly performed exercises out there, but when you get it right, they suddenly become very easy (and effective)! All you have to do is pretend like you're going to sit on a chair every time you bend your knees and lower your hips. Always sit back on your heels to make sure you're engaging your hamstrings and your glutes[24] (the backs of your legs and your butt muscles).

---

24   There are actually three gluteus muscles, the maximus, medius, and minimus. Fortunately, these bouncing squats with weights work all three of them simultaneously.

You should begin to do your Squats with just a gentle bounce, feet (or just heels) barely leaving the mat, or perhaps staying in contact with the mat the whole way through. As you become better and more stable at this, you can even extend the up-and-down of the squat to two or more bounce cycles at a time. Start slow, however. Get your back and leg muscles used to doing squats correctly before you get too fancy. You can also use handheld weights while you're doing squats like this, but first make sure your form is good, and then make sure you don't lose that good form as you add in the weights.

Handheld Weights Bouncing # 5: Triceps
Difficulty Level: Medium to high.
Special Emphasis or Benefits: Triceps, forearms.

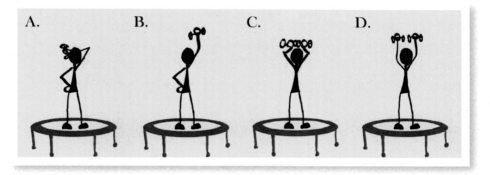

General Description: Working your triceps is essential to keeping your arms toned and strong. You want to be careful not to over-bend your elbows while performing these moves. Start small, slow...and light. The more you do these movements, the more your muscles will stretch and adapt as they get used to them, and the deeper you'll be able to go in each motion.

Variation # 1: Single Arm Overhead Triceps Extension (images A and B). Raise one of your arms over your head so that your elbow is almost behind your head. Bend your arms so that your weight is behind your head. Leaving your elbow and upper arm locked in place, extend your forearm so that your elbow straightens. Squeeze your tricep when your arm is straightest. Return to starting position.

Variation # 2: Overhead Triceps Extension with both arms (images C and D). This is a different motion than the one above, so please read these directions carefully. Begin with both arms straight overhead with your palms facing forward and arms shoulder width apart. Bend your elbows and lower your forearms behind you, making sure that your elbows and upper arms remain as stationary as possible. Keep your palms facing toward the sky or ceiling as you lower your arms as well. Straighten your arms and go back to the initial position. Alternatively, try this with a kettlebell once you're accustomed to the movement.

These, like every other handheld weight exercise on the rebounder, are great if you do them in rhythm to each of your bounces, up and down. Or you can slow it down so that your rhythm is one repetition to two bounces. This allows you to fully feel what gravity is doing and how heavy those weights are when they are in motion! And if it so happens that you can't really make it work to sync up or keep track of how many bounce cycles you're doing for each repetition of the exercise...well, just fuhgeddaboudit. Instead, just make sure (as always) that your posture is good, your breath is low and aware, and you're moving and grooving in a safe and sensible way.

B. Fast Bouncing and Running in Place

One of rebound exercise's unquestioned benefits is that it increases cardiovascular fitness through aerobic training. As we now know from decades of research on aerobic exercise, raising one's heart rate to a certain "target zone" is what makes the heart and lungs work harder and become stronger. Moreover, the entire concept of "interval training," which has received a good deal of attention, is based on cycles of vigorous movement. Moving vivaciously on your bouncer long enough each day is exactly what the doctor ordered.

Given the physics of rebounding generally, and the way that energy is re-circulated through the springs or bungee bands and mat, you can get yourself up to a powerful Fast Bouncing sequence pretty quickly. For example, you may be able to run in place as fast as you want for far longer than you ever could on hard ground without pounding your body to pieces. So go ahead, then, and take advantage of Fast Bouncing on your rebounder one or more times each workout session to increase bodily health and just have a good time. Listening to music with a fast driving beat is a great way to bounce fast. Fast Bouncing is also lots of fun and really gets your endorphins going.

Note that nearly any Bounce Type can be sped up to give you a good aerobic effect (see Appendix B). Here are three Bounce Type examples and variations for the Fast Bouncing Category:

1. Pulse Pace Flying
2. Pulse Pacing Back and Forth
3. Running in Place

Fast Bouncing # 1: Pulse Pace Flying
Difficulty Level: Medium.
Special Emphasis or Benefits: Easy way to raise your heart and respiration rates.

General Description: This is very similar to Pulsing in Place (found in the Easy Bouncing category), except here you use your arms to keep yourself pulsing at a fast pace, ideally to a musical beat. Typically your feet will stay on or close to the mat; that is, you will not rise very far off the mat, if at all. Your arms start near your sides and parallel with your thighs, and then trace an arc forward and up until they almost come together over your head with an almost "flapping" motion, as if you were a bird trying to take off. (You can also choose to only bring them as high as parallel with your shoulders if that's easier or more comfortable.) Your knees are slightly bent, your neck, shoulders, pelvis, and abdomen all as relaxed as possible (with the pelvis perhaps slightly tucked to promote a longer spine and more relaxed posture), and you might find yourself leaning forward a bit to keep everything balanced.

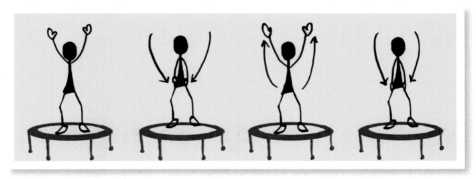

Comments: Pulse Pace Flying can be a lot of fun, especially to music. You can get yourself moving quite fast, up to 130 or 140 cycles per minute, if you're in reasonably good shape to start with and you work at it. This can be quite a sprint, so make sure you don't overdo it and exceed your maximum safe heart rate.

Variation # 1: Perform Pulse Pace Flying to a favorite fast song, the kind that you would normally only move to on every other beat, but instead move to it on every beat. Go ahead and challenge yourself aerobically, breathing in and out through your nose.

Variation # 2: Put a clock where you can see it and determine a set amount of time that you'll spend doing Pulse Pace Flying, such as one, two, or three minutes. If you have a favorite fast song you can use to set the pace here, then you can do one minute's worth, two minutes' worth, or more of that song. Jordan recommends David Bowie's classic "Suffragette City" for this.

Fast Bouncing # 2: Pulse Pacing Back and Forth
Difficulty Level: Medium.
Special Emphasis or Benefits: Another effective way to raise your heart rate; plus, you get some nice shoulder and back work.

General Description: This is also similar to Pulsing in Place from the Easy Bouncing category, except here you "throw" your arms all the way forward and then backward—behind your body—as you pulse up and down to a fast beat. You may find your body raising above and lowering into the mat a bit more here than with Pulsing in Place.

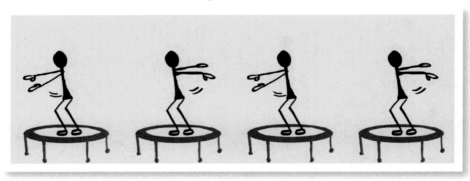

Comments: Pulse Pacing Back and Forth is also a lot of fun, especially to music. You can really "throw" yourself into (and out of) this particular bounce and get a very intense workout. Your arms, shoulders, and upper and mid back also receive a nice workout.

Variation # 1: Rather than moving your arms backward and forward, start out with your arms spread wide as shown below, bring them in horizontally until almost touching in front of you, then spread them out again. Keep your arms long and extended all the way through, but with soft elbows. In addition to aerobic benefits, you'll give your shoulder and chest muscles a good workout this way.

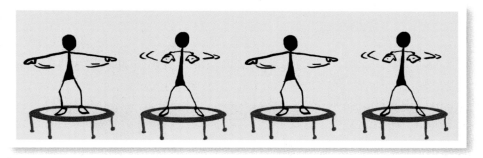

Fast Bouncing # 3: Running in Place
Difficulty Level: Medium to high.
Special Emphasis or Benefits: A great way to get moving and loosen your lower back.

General Description: Simply run in place. Move your arms to keep your balance, and pump them even harder when you want to pick up your pace. Work toward having your thighs come close to being parallel with the floor for at least some of each run. Start slowly and then pick up the pace as you get comfortable over time. Eventually, you can go very fast, and it can be a whole lot of fun.

Remember to keep your shoulders and neck relaxed and your pelvis and abs loose, and breathe in and out as fully and easily as you can. If you run out of breath, then slow down or do some other kind of Bounce Type as a transition until you regain your breath. You can also try breathing only through your nose while you run. This both increases your lung capacity and aligns your whole air intake system. Lastly, if you happen to hit a "glitch" in your gate—where your legs somehow miss a beat or you wobble or feel a "twang"—don't let this throw you off too much, as discussed in chapter 4. Make sure you're safe and unhurt, and then simply continue on.

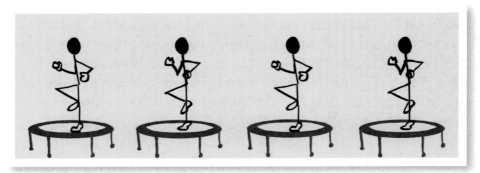

Comments: Running in Place not only offers a thorough aerobic workout, but as you alternately lift each leg, your lower back is given an opportunity to stretch out and relax.

Variation # 1: Use your clock to pick an amount of time that you will perform Running in Place, and then use a fast, fun song to set the pace.

Variation # 2: While holding light weights can be a lot of work, a lot of fun, and both exhilarating and exhausting. However, as discussed at length earlier, please be very careful when Running in Place to keep your light handheld weights light; that is, start with one-, two-, or at most three-pound handheld weights.

Avoid Running into a Rut

Running in Place becomes a prominent part of the basic bouncing repertoire for many people attracted to the Bounce. For those who once regularly ran on hard ground, but whose knees or other soft tissue can't tolerate this any longer, the possibility of long runs on a bouncer's giving surface is a bit of heaven. But be careful: don't be tempted to *only* Run in Place or let it dominate your entire practice.

Remember that the magic of the Bounce comes at least in part from how many different ways you're able to move your body while gravity surfing. Challenge yourself and don't get stuck in a rut doing the same few exercises over and over.

Instead, feel your body, listen to what it wants to do, and allow yourself to go there. And add in more movements and variations on top of whatever you're doing. Use your breath in mindful and creative ways, mix up the kinds of body movements and patterns you do, and you will soon be bouncing at or near your full personal potential.

C. High Bouncing

Bouncing far off the mat—rising high up into the air vertically—is invigorating, stimulating, and fun. For many, bouncing high is an essential—even necessary—part of bouncing, its very *raison d'être*. Certainly, when you're High Bouncing, you're doing something that you can pretty much only do safely on a rebounder (or a full-sized trampoline). There just aren't a lot of other ways to get the same "higher view" and sensation of rhythmically self-delivered flight in a safe, effective, delightful, and even exhilarating manner. After all, we're talking about flying here!

Common sense tells us that many of rebounding's undeniable benefits will be increased or amplified through High Bouncing. These benefits include increased lymph flow and therefore immune function, a stronger aerobic conditioning effect (bouncing higher is hard work), and increased core and leg strength, among others. Moreover, if you believe in the scientifically not-yet-proven claims made for rebound exercise that there is an "increased g-force effect"—where each of your cells is strengthened through its experience of going through first greater than, then lesser than, then greater than normal gravity—then bouncing as high as you can for at least some small part of each bouncing session becomes a desirable and perhaps essential component of rebound exercise.

Whether it's for physical health reasons or just for plain old fun, High Bouncing is something that many, if not most, people will want to try and perhaps include in their rebounding repertoire. If you're uncomfortable bouncing substantially high, then don't. It really isn't necessary for many or even most of rebound exercise's physical and metaphysical (emotional, spiritual, integral) benefits. On the other hand, you might be well advised to still occasionally go up to and perhaps a bit beyond your ordinary perceived height limits. You may find that you really like High Bouncing, even if you do it for only a short while each session.

The three Bounce Type examples (plus variations) provided for the High Bouncing category are:

1.   Just Bouncin' High
2.   Flyin' High
3.   Knee/Thigh Lift(off)—or "Kangaroo Jump"

High Bouncing # 1: Just Bouncin' High
Difficulty Level: Medium.
Special Emphasis or Benefits: Legs, core torso muscles, and balance.

General Description: As with Just Bouncin', there are times when you will want to bounce pretty high without having to think about it or make a big deal about it. Using mainly your core torso muscles to push down along with your lower legs to vigorously push off (from your toes through your calves), you can quite easily find yourself attaining some real altitude.

No particular arm movements or actions are necessary here. In fact, an important (and perhaps somewhat esoteric) aspect of Just Bouncin' High is learning how to completely relax so that you stay in the air, at the top of the bounce, for what at least subjectively feels like longer and longer periods of hang time. It may take some time to get the hang of this (ha ha), but it's well worth the effort.

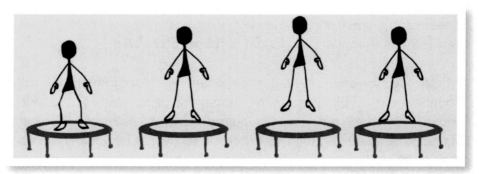

Comments: As with Just Bouncin', Just Bouncin' High is something that you can do at any time during a rebounding session. It works as a transition exercise between other bounces; it works if you're out of breath and need to switch to something else while your body reestablishes its respiratory equilibrium; and it works as its own focus if you're pursuing the sheer joy of gaining substantial vertical liftoff.

High Bouncing # 2: Flyin' High
Difficulty Level: Medium to high.
Special Emphasis or Benefits: Legs and core torso muscles, and shoulders and arms.

General Description: In Just Bouncin' High, the torso and legs were the primary drivers of the degree of liftoff achieved. Flyin' High adds in the arms; that is, since we don't have wings, we naturally try to fly with our arms. (You may have already gotten a taste of this in Pulse Pace Flying.) In fact, in addition to pushing down with core torso muscles and pushing off with calves and feet, you can think of yourself as pushing down with your arms to make yourself rise even higher.

Imagine, then, that the air is thick and offers resistance, and that by pushing down more forcefully, you can use the laws of physics to rise higher. Similarly, as you lift your arms up, the energy put into this motion causes you to rise higher as well. Note that you rise to the top of a bounce cycle both as your arms go down and as they go up.

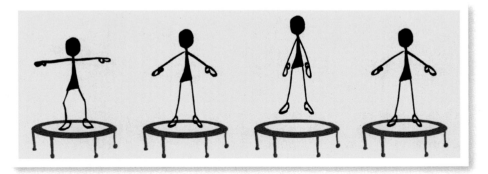

Comments: Note that the legs remain about the same distance apart throughout. At the top of the bounce, try to relax and extend your hang time.

Variation # 1: The "Power Pulse" adds a very forceful exhale at the bottom of the bounce, where you bring your arms down all the way. You can also bring your arms behind you and together as you forcefully exhale. You may not get quite as much height here as you do in the standard Flyin' High Bounce Type, but there is often a sense that the hang time at the top of the bounce is somehow increased both in proportion to the strength of forceful downward movement of the arms accompanying the exhale, and in proportion to how deeply you relax and just allow yourself to...float...at the top of the bounce.

High Bouncing # 3: Knee/Thigh Lift (Off!)—Kangaroo Jump
Difficulty Level: High. This Bounce Type is definitely not recommended for everybody.
Special Emphasis or Benefits: Uses thigh muscles to deliver sense of flight.

General Description: Although it's possible to get a sense of great height by lifting up your knees and thighs to jump off the rebounder mat, this Bounce Type is not recommended for most people. It can be hard to stay in control for more than one or at most two bounces, because so much of the body's weight first is lifted so high and then comes back down with a great deal of force. If you're going to experiment with this Bounce Type, start relatively low and mellow, and then work your way up higher.

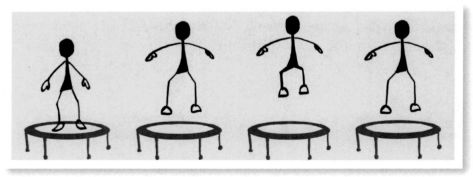

Comments: This type of bounce is reminiscent of the way a kangaroo jumps off the ground. In fact, it is more like jumping than it is like bouncing. Because it fully engages some of the body's largest muscle groups, incorporating a few of these into your routine once you feel "up" to it (ha ha) can really take your workout up a notch. However, for some and possibly many people, this Bounce Type can be truly hard to safely control for any type of long or extended sequence (or even for a single bounce cycle). Go low and slow at first, especially if you have any lower back issues, and really make sure that you're good with the basic movement before you get too far (and high) into it.

‖ D. Slow Bouncing

Slow Bouncing doesn't have any subcategories, because it is itself a kind of subcategory. The idea here is easy: Take nearly any previous bounce discussed in this chapter, except movements that are all about being fast (like Fast Bouncing), and then go ahead and slow it down...way...w...a...y... down. In fact, go ahead and do whatever it is—Jumping Jacks, twists, pulsing in place—just as slowly, methodically, and purposefully as you possibly can. Keep your movements strong and stay conscious of your breath as you really feel into your body, and you give yourself the luxurious experience of going very slow.

Obviously, if you slow down too far, you'll lose momentum, your form will stutter and break, and at a certain point you won't really be bouncing at all. So keep it just a notch above that, and you'll find that there are many challenges and opportunities—many opportunities for learning—that simply do not present themselves at higher speeds. Balance and strength, in particular, rise to the forefront in terms of what you'll be focusing on and working with when you slow way, way down.

A few quick tips on Slow Bouncing for you:

- Make sure you keep breathing well, with a functional awareness of your breath the whole way through, and since you're going slow, you can probably stick with both inhaling and exhaling through your nose.
- If you find yourself on the verge of falling off, or of losing momentum entirely, then speed things up just a tick.
- As always, heed your body and any warning signs of danger: excess pain, fear of falling off, and so on.

Type 3: Advanced and Specialized Bounces

‖ A. Cross-Legged Bouncing

Difficulty Level: Medium to high.

Special Emphasis or Benefits: This movement can be physically challenging for the feet, legs, calves, and thighs as well as the pelvis and lower back. It can also be neurologically challenging and stimulating; that is, since it's something your brain doesn't expect, it's typically experienced as novel and interesting.

General Description: Cross-Legged Bouncing involves doing something that is pretty simple and simultaneously complex and potentially very difficult. You "simply" cross one foot and leg in front of the other, and then stay that way and bounce (see Variation 1) or cross and uncross your legs over time (Variation 2). After we go through Cross-Legged Bouncing once, we're going to give you even more detail and analysis of exactly what's going on here, and some additional options you can try.

Comments: It's important to start slow with Cross-Legged Bouncing. Specifically, when you first try Variation 1, keep your feet mostly or completely on the mat, perhaps letting your heels rise off a little bit. Stay aware of your breathing the whole way through, and maintain good posture throughout the movement.

Variation # 1: Here you cross one foot in front of or behind the other, and leave them crossed that way for a set number of repetitions as you lightly bounce up and down. You don't need much or any vertical takeoff here, and your feet can stay mostly or completely in contact with the mat. When you're done with doing it one way, uncross your feet and legs for a few bounces, and then immediately cross your feet and legs the other way and do the same number of repetitions. Note that the more you bend your knees, the more challenging the movement becomes. If you can't keep your posture good and your breath low, strong, and steady, then you're bending your knees too far.

Variation # 2: This is more difficult, so start slow (and if you're using music, do it to slow music). Let's say that each time your feet hit the mat, or each time your weight goes down into the bottom of the mat, it counts as one beat. Start out in a neutral position, with your legs shoulder width apart. Then, on the first beat, you want to cross one leg over the other. On the second beat, you want to bring your legs back out to a normal bouncing position. Then, on the third beat, you want to cross your legs the *other* way (if your right foot was in front, then your left foot will now be in front). Then, on the fourth beat, go back to neutral. (Note that while it's possible to swing your legs around on every other beat, without taking advantage of going back to a neutral position, doing so is much more difficult and could possibly even lead to injury.)

Variation # 3: Add in Jumping Jacks while you're doing either Variation # 1 (feet and legs stay in same crossed position for a certain number of reps) or Variation # 2 (feet and legs cross back and forth over time).

Variation # 4: Same as Variation # 3, but add in light handheld weights with your Jumping Jacks.

Additional Details and Analysis on Cross-Legged Bouncing: There are a variety of factors you can use to vary and enhance your Cross-Legged Bouncing, including how far behind or in front of you the leg and foot you're moving go. Suppose you have a stable leg and foot, which stay on or near the center of your rebounder mat, and a mobile leg and foot that do the actual crossing, so to speak. Your mobile foot can fall 45 degrees in front of or behind the other foot, or can be directly lined up behind or in front of it, or even go around it, most of the way up to a full semicircle.

Consider the following diagram. Suppose you begin with your left foot, labeled as A, as the stable leg and foot that start out and stay in the middle of the rebounder. B represents your right foot in the starting neutral position. C shows your mobile right foot at roughly a 45-degree angle. D shows your right foot directly in front of your left foot, and E shows it coming nearly all the way around, most of the way to a full semicircle. In position C you're just starting to do cross-legged bouncing, and then you're fully doing it in position D, and position E represents an even more extended stretch, where you have brought your mobile foot most of the way around.

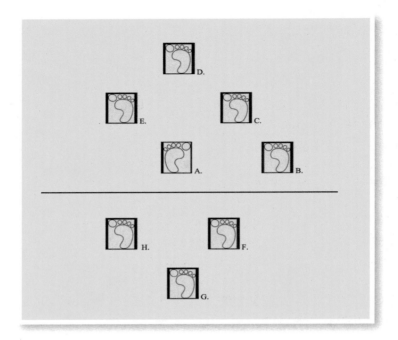

- In Variation # 2, described above, you can experiment with both how many times you bounce with your legs crossed on each side, and how many times you bounce in the neutral middle position.
- In all Cross-Legged Bouncing, you can vary how much you bend your knees. The more you bend your knees, the more difficult it becomes, especially with regard to your knees and back. As always, let pain be your guide and don't overdo it.
- Finally, you should be aware that you really have four, not two, major options: If your right foot is the one doing the active crossing, as shown in the diagram above, then as you start out, it can move either in front of your left foot (as in positions C, D, and E), or behind your stable foot, as in positions F, G, and H. You may *think* that moving your left foot behind your right foot is pretty much going to be exactly the same thing as moving your right foot in front of your left foot—but in reality, they are very different movements that will affect your body very differently. That is, the leg and foot (along with everything attached to them) that stay stable and in the center will be activated and challenged in very different ways depending on whether your mobile foot crosses in front of your

stationary foot or behind it. Go ahead and try it—very slowly at first—and you'll see what we mean.

B. Structured Strength in Motion™ (SSiM™)

Difficulty Level: Medium to high.
Special Emphasis or Benefits: There are many different ways to do SSiM, and almost any part of your body can be challenged or benefited when doing this kind of movement.

General Description: SSiM is somewhat difficult to explain and illustrate, but once you "get it," you'll be glad to have it as part of your repertoire. Here, you tense, freeze, or "lock out" some portion of your body—your arms, your entire upper torso, your legs, your upper torso and legs, and so on—and you hold that position while moving up and down. Even with attention placed on the breath, and the relaxation of those parts of the body not being purposefully held in place, it can take a tremendous amount of focus and strength to bounce in this way.

In effect, you have created a structure[25] (the parts of you that are tensed) that takes a good deal of strength to hold in position, especially while you're in motion—hence, Structured Strength in Motion. The image below illustrates a very simple example of SSiM focused on holding the arms raised up and to the side while keeping the feet, legs, and torso in the same position throughout.

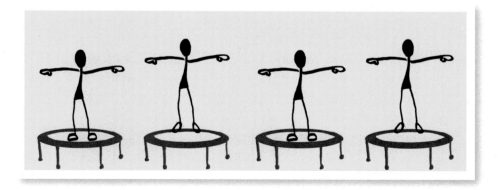

---

25 Chapter 8's discussion of the body as a "tensegrity structure" is relevant here.

Comments: SSiM is really more of a feeling to be experienced than an exact set of physical positions or instructions that can be conveyed in words or even pictures. Don't limit yourself here. There is practically no limit to the variations that you can come up with, as this is a very free-form process.

To create your own SSiM movements: (1) find a position in which you want to develop additional strength, (2) hold the engaged body parts and structures where they are as you bounce, and (3) keep breathing into and through the entire physical and energetic pattern that you have formed with your body. If things become too intense, a slight change in position may enable you to work through whatever it is that is going on, similar to the Work-It-Through Bounce Type in the Breathwork Category.

Loosen Up and Let Go:
A Comment on Structured Strength in Motion™

Ed Lark, of Sebastopol, California, is a master teacher and practitioner of massage and bodywork. Over a decade ago, Jordan described to him some of the things that he'd experienced while bouncing, including Breathwork Bouncing, Bodywork Bouncing, and SSiM, and asked him if he had any insights about just how it might be possible for pain to "loosen up" and go away with focused bouncing.

Ed's response was that in a manner similar to the Trager® massage method, which involves very light, gentle, rhythmic shaking movements, it was his guess that rebounding worked to mechanically and neurologically over-stimulate and thereby trigger tissue changes through sensory-motor feedback loops between the muscles and brain. Then, in a kind of "what the heck" reaction, the muscles and other tissue find themselves relaxing, reorganizing, and balancing out.

"What you're saying," Jordan replied, "is that rebounding works to shake out and loosen disharmonious, painful, and poorly connected 'stuff' in the body—is that right?"

"That's it," Ed said. "You've got it."

C. Abdominal and Stretch Bouncing

In this section, we'll discuss both Abdominal Bouncing and Stretch Bouncing.

Abdominal Bouncing: 3 Variables
Difficulty Level: Medium to hard.
Special Emphasis or Benefits: Tones abs, builds core strength, and challenges the lower back.

You may have seen images of a young man with incredibly chiseled abs lying on his back on a rebounder, legs held out straight, arms pulsing up and down to work his core. We're not quite clear that anyone has ever achieved such abs only through Abdominal Bouncing on their back like this, but we can say that it is one heck of a workout and probably can't hurt—unless you do it improperly, in an unbalanced way, or for too long, in which case, as with nearly everything else in life and in the Bounce, you can indeed hurt yourself.

In addition to staying fully present with your breath, the three main variables here are:

- **Quantity:** How long can you keep your form good and still keep pulsing? You can measure the quantity of time on the clock ("Yeah! I kept going for 60 whole seconds!"), or just in terms of how many pulses you do with good form (25, 50, 100?—just how badly do you want those chiseled abs?).
- **Angle of your legs:** Forty-five degrees seems to be the hardest angle to hold. You can raise your legs up, or lower them down, to adjust the intensity of your abs work.
- **Angle of arm spread:** You can hold both arms directly in front of you, pointing forward and mimicking your legs, or you can open them up so that they are at a 45-degree angle coming out of your body, or totally outstretched to the side. How far you spread out your arms will affect which back, shoulder, arm, and core muscles are being used to do your pulsing.

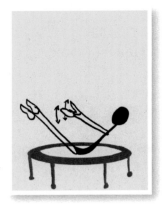
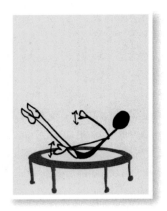

Stretch Bouncing # 1: Back Bends
Difficulty Level: Medium.
Special Emphasis or Benefits: Opens up the lower, mid, and upper back.

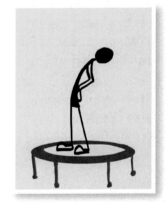

General Description: Place your hands on your lower back and gently and slowly lower yourself backward as far as you are comfortable, then try Pulsing in Place, Just Bouncin', or any other simple bounce.

Comments: Back bends of all types are a staple of modern yoga as they can do an excellent job of releasing the back and opening the whole body. But you obviously don't want to go too far, especially at first, and if you feel pain or at all dizzy, you should of course stop. Place attention on the breath, as always, and make sure you keep your head and shoulders, as well as your pelvis and abdomen, as relaxed as possible. Come up slowly, and do some transitional bounces or Breathwork Bouncing before going on.

Stretch Bouncing # 2: Front Bends
Difficulty Level: Medium.
Special Emphasis or Benefits: Good stretch for
lower back, hip flexors, calves, and hamstrings.

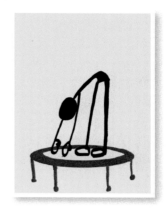

General Description: Stand on the rebounder,
bend your knees as much as you need to, and
reach down and place the palms of your hand
on the mat. Then move up and down as if you
were Pulsing in Place, with your palms and feet
staying on the mat.

Comments: The key thing to watch here is
moving your head too quickly, especially when
you come up from this position. If you're dizzy,
then try some type of basic transition bounce
(e.g., Just Bouncin' or simple Jumping Jacks),
until you have reached equilibrium. You can get
a really good stretch here, but you always have
to move slowly and be extra careful.

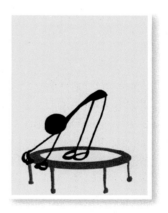

Variation # 1: Hold on to the outside frame of
the rebounder instead of placing your hands on
the mat to stretch your back. Dig your heels into the mat and allow the
flex of the mat to increase the stretch in your calves.

Variation # 2: Place your knuckles instead of the palms of your hands
on the mat.

Stretch Bouncing # 3: Child's Resting Pose
Difficulty Level: Easy.
Special Emphasis or Benefits: Stretches out the legs and the lower back.

General Description: Anyone who has done even a little bit of yoga will
be familiar with the Child's Pose, also known as the Child's Resting Pose
("Balasana" in Sanskrit). Essentially, you kneel on the rebounder, with your
upper body folded on top of your lower body (your chest folded onto your

thighs). Note that depending on your knee, hip, and back flexibility, this may be hard for you, and you may not be able to go all the way down. If you can comfortably get some or most of the way down, do some deep breathing in this position, with your arms either in front of you, perhaps holding on to the rim of the rebounder, or tucked against your sides and behind you.

Variation # 1: Once you're down and relaxed, try pulsing up and down a little, breathing into any tight or restricted places in your body.

Stretch Bouncing # 4: Squat Pulses
Difficulty Level: Medium.
Special Emphasis or Benefits: Great for stretching out the hips, back, and hamstrings.

General Description: Stand on the rebounder and place your hands on your thighs as you squat down a bit. Then bounce up and down as if you were Pulsing in Place. Your feet can stay entirely on the mat, your heels can come off the mat, or you can go ahead and gain some altitude as you pulse. Keep your back flat and head, face, and neck relaxed.

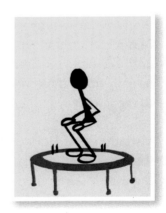

Comments: This is a great movement for the lower back as well as the thighs and buttocks. By placing your hands on your thighs, you mostly "lock out" the upper body and the emphasis turns to stretching and balance. But be particularly careful here not to move your head around too much; once again, you want your head—although fluid and loose—to remain stable and mostly in one position.

Variation # 1: Place your hands on your knees rather than your thighs. This changes the angle of the body and can enable you to "lock out" and hold your upper body in some very different ways, thereby giving yourself a wider variety of back stretches.

‖ *D. One-Legged Bouncing*

Difficulty Level: Extremely high; **not recommended** for your first year of bouncing.
Special Emphasis or Benefits: Leg strength and balance.

We weren't sure about discussing one-legged bouncing in this book. We decided that specific instruction on it was best saved for a future work. Even Jordan, who has been bouncing now for nearly 18 years, finds one-legged bouncing fairly challenging and demanding (especially 50 repetitions on each leg, with arms added to imitate the Hindu religion's Dancing Shiva or Shiva Nataraja). So our advice is this:

Don't even think of trying one-legged bouncing until you have at least a year of regular bouncing behind you. It's just too easy for things to go wrong, and as always, safety must come first.

Layering and Gearing

Throughout this chapter, we often advise you to start slowly, doing just one thing at a time. But as you gain more experience and confidence, as you become stronger and more flexible over time, you will likely be drawn to doing things that are more complex as well as more intense.

It's relatively easy to move up the complexity scale through what we call *layering*. This simply means adding another layer of movement or some other discrete activity on top of what you're already doing. So, for example, suppose you're doing simple Jumping Jacks, and it's going fine, but you want to do something more. Well, you can cross your arms at the top of the bounce, with your right hand going in front of your left. Then you can practice your left hand going in front of your right. Then you can alternate, right hand in front of left, then left hand in front of right. By doing this, you have added a couple of new layers.

But wait! Why stop there? You can also start crossing your legs and feet every bounce cycle or every two bounce cycles. And then, perhaps, you can add in very light handheld weights (perhaps first using them without crossing your hands, and then re-adding the crossing motion). And then, on top of all that, you can layer on some breathwork, perhaps doing a three-three-three-three pattern (inhale for three pulses, hold in for three, exhale for three, hold out for three).

Not only are there almost always new layers to add on top of *whatever* Bounce Type, sequence, or movement you're already doing, but you'll find that doing so is fun, interesting, and neuro-physiologically exciting and stimulating. Let's replay what was just described so you can see how it adds up to something entirely more complex and interesting over time:

- Layer 1: Simple Jumping Jacks
- Layer 2: Jumping Jacks with arms crossing, left in front of right
- Layer 3: Jumping Jacks with arms crossing, right in front of left
- Layer 4: Jumping Jacks with arms crossing alternately, left then right in front
- Layer 5: Jumping Jacks with arms crossing alternately, with feet crossing as well
- Layer 6: Jumping Jacks with arms crossing alternately with feet crossing as well, while holding light handheld weights
- Layer 7: Everything that's come before, but adding breathwork on top of it

If you go ahead and try this sequence, you'll see that each new successive layer changes up the whole experience. This has the effect of causing you to be more fully present, and as a result, additional wonderful things—like moving into flow states—can more readily happen. Keep in mind, then, that a new layer can consist of:

- Doing something additional with your arms and shoulders
- Doing something additional with your feet or legs
- Doing something additional with an accessory, like handheld weights
- Doing something additional that is mainly internal, like breath counting

- Doing something additional like singing or chanting
- Doing something additional with just your hands and fingers

In addition to layering, we also like to think in terms of *gearing*. You'll notice that each successive layer in the above example may or may not be more intense than the previous layer. For example, moving from layer 2 to layer 3 is no more intense, and moving from layer 6 to layer 7, while taking additional mental energy, is also no more physically intense. On the other hand, moving from layer 4 to 5, which brings in the crossing of feet, is probably going to be more intense, and moving to layer 6, where you have added light handheld weights, will almost certainly be more intense.

As opposed to *layering,* with *gearing* the focus is on intensity. By analogy to a car or even a bicycle, you move into a higher gear by increasing your energetic intensity and work output as you move faster, bounce higher, or use heavier weights. Suppose you are in layer 4 of the above example, with your feet remaining essentially flat and staying in contact with the mat the whole way through—and now you want to gear up.

The first thing to do—while continuing to do Jumping Jacks and cross your arms—might be to lift your heels off the mat with each movement. Not much of a gear increase, but a little. Then you could gear up a little more by lifting all of both your feet a little bit off the mat each time. Next, you gear up even more by putting a substantial amount of energy in and bouncing pretty high off the mat each time. You're doing the same thing, but you've moved into a higher gear.

Or consider running in place to a fast song. Go ahead and put on David Bowie's "Suffragette City," and run pretty slow to it. Then go ahead and gear up and find a medium pace that will keep you in sync with the music. And then, if you want, gear up to full-intensity running, trying to match Bowie's beat even when it gets fast. Same movement, same song, but a variety of different gears to experience it through.

If you keep *layering* and *gearing* in mind, you'll *never* run out of new and interesting ways to experience the Bounce. You'll always be able to change things around, adding a little of this, substituting a little of that, ramping up or down your intensity (*gearing* down as well as *gearing* up), and overall creating a wild variety of possible movement sequences for any given rebounding session.

The best way to use this chapter's Compendium is one Bounce Type at a time, one layer at a time, one gear at a time. If you take to the Bounce, you have a lifetime of exploration ahead of you.

Section III:

Advanced Bouncing, and the 45 X 45 Challenge

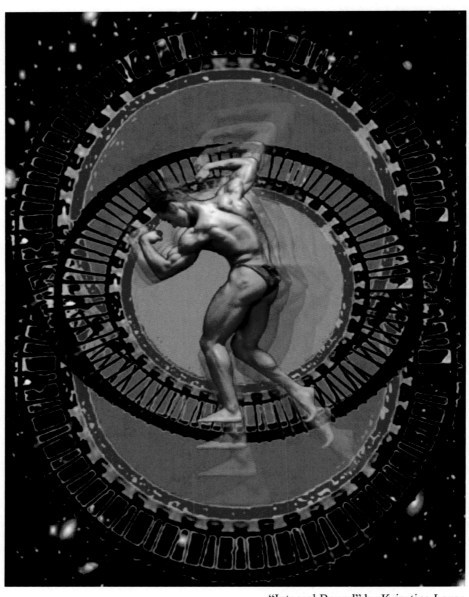

"Integral Bound" by Krisztina Lazar

Chapter 6:

Spiritual/Inner Work:
Tools and Practices

So far we've focused mostly on the Bounce's physical benefits, convenience, and fun, easy nature. But there's another dimension—an inner dimension—that's just as important to our lives. The question then becomes how to best integrate body, mind, and spirit as we bring our favorite inner work and play to bouncing.

We've found that rebounding provides a ready opportunity for the empowering discovery of some wonderful inner experiences and states of mind. Bouncing, all by itself, can bring you to bliss and immerse you in what's been called *flow*. If you then combine your bouncing with the knowledge, tools, or techniques of any number of spiritual or human development traditions, then truly wonderful things—spiritual things, mystical things, magical things, transcendent things—can happen.

This chapter will therefore begin with some psycho-spiritual overview material, and then present a smorgasbord of spiritual and self-development tools and ideas. We trust that as our curious and intelligent reader, you'll explore as many of these ideas and techniques as you're comfortable with. Always keep in mind that there's no required creed or technique—and certainly no one way—when it comes to exploring the psychological opportunities and spiritual benefits of rebound exercise. This is another area where we both welcome and expect many outside experts to contribute ideas and practices.

If you already have a spiritual or self-development practice of some kind, then go ahead and bring it to your time on the rebounder. Or, if it just so happens that the psycho-spiritual domain and toolset explored in this chapter doesn't appeal to you, we're absolutely fine with that too. Bouncing will still be good for you on the inside!

However this chapter resonates for you, we invite you to peruse it with an open mind. Be pragmatic but also empirical as you experiment

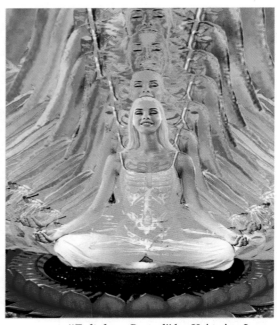

"Enlighten Bound" by Krisztina Lazar

with what's presented here. You have a lot to gain, very little to lose, and a big wide inner world to experience and explore!

Rebounding Naturally Invites and Brings About Inner Work

One of the truly wonderful things about bouncing is that, in addition to addressing the needs of the physical body in a powerful and effective way, it both offers the opportunity to do inner work and tends to automatically bring it about.

The opportunity is both obvious and to a certain degree inescapable. Having established a regular rebound exercise practice, you'll find yourself there on the rebounder, bouncing up and down, for some amount of time each day or nearly each day. What are you going to do with all that time? Listening to music or podcasts, watching TV, and talking on a phone headset, as discussed earlier, are effective time-passing options.

But in an age of nearly infinite distractions, it's clearly better to not occupy ourselves *all of the time* with external inputs. Even if you love music or TV, sometimes you'll want a break, to give yourself the opportunity to fully experience the Bounce with no external distractions. (Of course, you can also do inner work with good music on.)

So again, there you are, bouncing up and down, using your body in ways that are more or less simple or complicated, easy or intense, depending on the day, your time window, your intention, and your energy level. As you gain mastery over basic bounces, movements, and accessory equipment, there will be moments when you'll have enough free attention to go inward if you choose to. And not only will you have the opportunity, but the very act of bouncing may induce you to go inward in two distinct ways.

The first way has to do with the repetitive, trance-inducing nature of the activity itself.

Some might find rebounding's natural rhythm repetitive and boring, but most people seem to experience it as soothing, somewhat hypnotic, and capable of putting them into a light trance or slightly altered state of mind. Thus, through the ancient method of repetitive trance-inducing motion, rebounding can open the doorway to certain types of inner work and vision.

The second way is a kind of big-picture effect—perhaps a meta-level impact—that comes from how well rebound exercise addresses the physical body. You see, when your body knows it's being well taken care of—when you become aware you are actually powerfully addressing your own physical needs in real time—it becomes much easier to relax, come fully present, and give yourself the opportunity to do whatever kind of inner work you might need, want, or benefit from. That is, the more we know for certain that we're being lovingly physically nurtured, the better we feel and the more we are drawn to taking advantage of the full spectrum of our inner resources.

As both psychologist Abraham Maslow and economist Karl Marx have said in their own way, you have to address the physical substratum or level of our lives first, and then you can move up the ladder of needs, desires, goals, and actualization. As one friend of ours who has embraced the Bounce likes to say: "When I'm bouncing, I feel that my body is okay. That I'm okay. And that makes me feel really good."

As you're not going anywhere anyway, the Bounce really does offer you a splendid ongoing inner opportunity. It also offers you two ways in. It has an inherently trance-inducing nature, plus it frees up your energy so you can focus internally. The question then becomes: "What kind of inner work should I do? What will work best for me? What's available, and how do I even go about it?"

How to Approach Bringing Spiritual Tools and Techniques to Bouncing

If you already have a spiritual practice or do some kind of inner work, see if it naturally and obviously transposes onto the rebounder. Let's use meditation as an example. While some forms of meditation strictly require the meditator to sit still, there are many types of moving meditations that can be done while you're rebounding. You might find it hard to make it work, or it might turn out to be a natural and easy transposition. Give it a try, see what happens, take some notes, and decide if it's worth trying it again.

If you're not already doing some kind of regular inner spiritual work or practice, then perhaps pick something you've heard about that sounds interesting, or go with something you tried in the past and liked, but gave up on for one reason or another. Perhaps the Bounce will help you experience whatever it was in a fresh, new way. Or you might decide to pick one of the techniques or modes of inner work from the following list and try it out while bouncing.

Almost every one of the tools or options for inner work listed below is, in and of itself, a huge topic that has been extensively expounded on by many teachers, books, and websites. It won't be hard for you to find information on almost anything suggested here, and there are many, many more options out there that we haven't listed.

Bottom line: the Bounce offers you a fantastic opportunity to do inner work. But it's up to you to choose which kind, to find out about it, and to then apply it to your bouncing time. If you like what you're doing—if it's producing real behavioral and other desirable changes in your world—there may be times when you find your inner work taking up most or even all of a bouncing session. And that's just fine, because as long as you're moving your body and bouncing during that time, you'll be receiving many, if not most, of the physical benefits that rebound exercise so readily offers.

An Alphabetical List of Inner/Spiritual Tools and Practices for Bouncing

Here's a short alphabetical list of inner work choices that may be adaptable to rebounding:

- *Breathwork* can be as simple as counting your breaths (for example, in for three, hold for three, out for three, hold out for three) or doing more advanced breathing techniques (in for four, hold for seven, out for eight)—but if you get dizzy, you're doing too much.
- *Chakra* visualization and invocation involves seeing and sensing flows of energy moving in and through the seven chakras.[26]
- *Chanting* or *singing* can be spiritually oriented chants, songs, or anything you like that engages the voice.
- *Juggling* may at first seem a bit surprising to include in a list of inner work. Well, juggling on a rebounder takes quite a bit of concentration and focus. Give it a try. (We haven't seen many people succeed at this, actually, so take it as a dare. Just too many variables in play even for proficient jugglers.)
- *Kabbalah* visualizations and invocations, such as doing Pathwork or otherwise centering in individual charkas or "inner worlds" and moving through them.

---

26 To learn more about the chakras, read Anodea Juidth's bestselling 1987 work, *Wheels of Life.*

- *Kundalini* yoga includes many exercises having to do with breath, mudra, and body position that can be readily adapted to rebounding.
- *Mandalas*, like Tibetan thangkas, yantras, and prayer flags allow us to take a deep dive into visually arresting religious imagery and geometric patterns.
- *Mantras* such as "Om Mani Padme Hum," associated with specific Eastern traditions or deities—or a modern one you make up for yourself—are very relaxing and beneficial when repeated over and over again.
- *Martial arts* movements and meditations done on a rebounder can help strengthen both the inner and outer aspects of your martial arts practice as well as your bouncing practice. For example, Tai Chi can be easy to engage in while bouncing.
- *Meditation* can be as simple as clearing your mind and not thinking. A sense-anchored mindfulness meditation practice can easily be undertaken by just noting when your feet are—or are not—in contact with the mat.
- *Mudras*—holding specific hand and finger positions—are designed to create energy flows and trigger states of consciousness.
- *Oracular* bouncing involves taking a question about your life or the future and holding it in your mind all the way through your bounce time. Sometimes, an answer will be "revealed" or will otherwise come to you.
- *Prayer*, from any tradition—or entirely homegrown—is perfect for bouncing.
- *Sufi*-type bouncing would include twirling and many other forms of dance (e.g., Dances of Universal Peace), hand motions, and so on that can potentially be brought to the bouncer. (But be very careful if you twirl!)

Feeling Like You're Floating and Flying

Something truly exceptional seems to happen at the top of each bouncing cycle. There may be some good physiological, neurological, or psychological reasons for this, or it may just be an artifact of weightlessness experienced by the stomach. In any case, learning to extend at least the subjective if not objective experience of one's hang time can be very rewarding and is a worthwhile challenge.

It's unlikely that any of us will ever duplicate basketball great Michael Jordan's talents here, but by "bouncing big" and then completely relaxing at the top, it may be possible to extend our hang time. And while most of us have never had the kind of flow Michael Jordan regularly produced at the highest level of athletic performance, almost all of us at some point or other in our lives have had experiences of athletic flow performance beyond what we're normally capable of.

So just for fun, make it your intention to increase your hang time, and do this at a point in your session when you're already well into the flow of the Bounce. You just might surprise yourself with at least the subjective experience of "floating" or "flying" that you can bring about here.

The Bounce as an Integral Transformative Practice

Rebound exercise embodies many of the qualities of what has been called "Integral Transformative Practice" or ITP. In their wonderful book *The Life We Are Given* (1995), George Leonard and Michael Murphy lay out the notion of an ITP—a practice that deals with body, mind, heart, and soul. An ITP is aimed at positive changes in inner and outer well-being. And it involves a *practice*, that is, something that you do in a long-term, disciplined manner and that has value in and of itself.

Not only does bouncing powerfully and effectively address the body, it invites and even induces the performance of inner work, as described above. Moreover, bouncing works best when it's done as a regular practice, on a daily or near-daily basis.

As we often point out, not only is bouncing fun, but for quite a few people it's downright joyful and even ecstatic. In a certain sense, every time we bounce we are literally—actually—getting high (and then low), and every time we bounce, we are figuratively connecting Heaven and Earth. In this way, a committed practice of the Bounce can serve as the cornerstone of your own ITP. Another way to get to your own ITP is through the Vitruvian Super Self model, which we'll turn to now.

The Vitruvian Super Self— Moving and Grooving in 4D

Let's begin to imagine ourselves as Leonardo da Vinci's iconic Vitruvian Man, which for our purposes we'll rename the Vitruvian Human. Leonardo drew this iconic image while he was working with the mathematician Luca Pacioli. He was studying the proportional theories of Vitruvius, a 1st-century Roman architect. Imposing the principles of geometry on the human body, Leonardo illustrated Vitruvius' theory by showing that when a man places his feet on the ground, he can be contained in the lines of a square, but when in spread-eagle position, he fits perfectly in a circle. According to the *Encyclopaedia Britannica*:[27]

> Leonardo envisaged the great picture chart of the human body he had produced through his anatomical drawings and *Vitruvian Man* as a *cosmografia del minor mondo* (cosmography of the microcosm). He believed the workings of the human body to be an analogy, in microcosm, for the workings of the universe. Leonardo wrote: "Man has been called by the ancients a lesser world, and indeed the name is well applied; because, as man is composed of earth, water, air, and fire...this body of the earth is similar."

"Cosmography of the microcosm"—the workings of the human body are an analogy for the workings of the universe! Everything is connected. Your body is reflected in the earth. As above, so below. These ideas convey the simple but profound truth that as human beings, we are a mirror of the environment and universe around us, necessarily and inescapably interconnected to both.

---

27   See http://www.britannica.com/biography/Leonardo-da-Vinci.

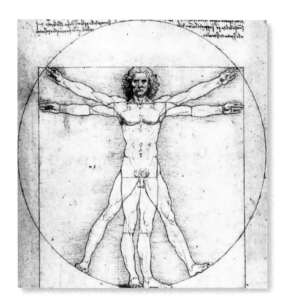

Like the yolk within an egg, we're a part of something larger than us, but something that is inextricably also "us" as well. Thus, the Sun is part of the solar system, which is part of the galaxy, which is part of the universe; similarly, an atomic nucleus is part of an atom, which is part of a molecule, which is part of a cell, which is part of an organ, which is part of our body. (The integral philosopher Ken Wilber, following in the footsteps of the great Arthur Koestler, calls this "holons within holons"; that is, parts that are within wholes that are in turn parts of larger wholes, all the way up to the largest cosmological structures of the universe, and all the way down to the smallest subatomic particles.[28])

Think about all these kinds of relationships. What do you notice about them? Your brain creates an image of what we're referring to, and it all seems to be best depicted as something that is roughly spherical or ovoid in nature. Look at the Vitruvian Human: they're inside a circle. This shape is intrinsic to understanding "wholeness" because it best represents the idea of completion, with no sharp corners or disruptions of form.

Please ponder a circle for a moment (see below). Trace the shape with your mind, following its endless curve all the way around the outside circumference. Examine the unbrokenness of its shape and continue to

---

28   See https://en.wikipedia.org/wiki/Holon_%28philosophy%29.

trace the line that has no beginning and no end with your mind's eye. Feel what that shape does to your body and to your breath as you continue to meditate on it. It's no wonder that in many spiritual, mystical, and religious systems, as well as systems of health and healing, the circle represents unsullied origins and unbroken wholeness.

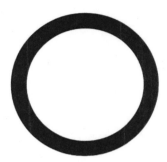

When you're ready, move your awareness into the third dimension and meditate for a moment on a circle now turned into a *sphere* (below). Investigate the outside of the sphere with your mind. Feel how the circle has transformed, and follow the unbroken multidimensional surface of the sphere. Inhabit and feel the shape of the sphere with your senses, and attempt to fully understand what it means to be uninterrupted, whole, and extended in this way. Now, notice how you feel. Check in gently with your emotions and bring awareness to what is going through your mind, and really notice how you're feeling.

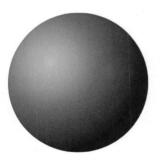

Do you perhaps feel a little better than a few minutes ago, just by thinking of this shape? If so, then this is pretty powerful stuff. We believe that the contemplation of wholeness is extraordinarily healing all by itself;

it is essentially what mandalas the world over are used for. But what if instead of just *thinking* about a sphere, you could BE one, could move your body to BECOME one? What if you, yourself—your body—could become a three-dimensional mandala[29] moving through time?

Begin by picturing a bubble around your body. Imagine that you're surrounded by an aura made of energy, but instead of it being a static egg around your body, it's a dynamic flow of energy that reacts to your intentions. It moves with you and responds to you. The energy invigorates you and is simultaneously invigorated by you. You can touch the outside of it with your fingertips. As you move your body, you begin to manipulate its shape and intensity, "filling in" your energy sphere with ever more complex spokes, swirls, and montages of your own personal and unique cosmic mandala.

There are many traditions and shamans that describe an energy field that radiates almost spherically around you. You might remember Carlos Castaneda describing an egg-shaped luminous aura surrounding the body in his books:

> Our total being consists of two perceivable segments. The first is the familiar physical body, which all of us can perceive; the second is the luminous body, which is a cocoon that only seers can perceive, a cocoon that gives us the appearance of giant luminous eggs.
>
> One of the most important goals of sorcery is to reach the luminous cocoon; a goal which is fulfilled through the sophisticated use of *dreaming* and through a rigorous, systematic exertion called *not-doing*. I've defined not-doing as an unfamiliar act which engages our total being by forcing it to become conscious of its luminous segment.[30]

Instead of sorcery the way Castaneda or his teacher Don Juan might have described it, with bouncing we are reaching out to and working with our

---

29   Mandalas range from the very simple to the very complex, and many mystical and spiritual practitioners begin their meditations with the simplest form of mandala, the circle, or with a more complex elaboration of a circle.

30   See http://www.prismagems.com/castaneda/donjuan6.html.

own luminous cocoons through a type of self-propelled wizardry of our own making. Opening up the channels of movement in a physical, visceral, multidimensional way is magical in its own right. In the flow of the Bounce, you're moving in ways that engage and even fully awaken your total being. In this way, bouncing energizes, expands, and makes terrific use of the great scope and power of our mind-body connection.

What differentiates bouncing from nearly any other terrestrial-based activity (with swimming a standout exception) is that you can relatively easily move your body through space in lots of different ways and configurations—up and down, side to side, in and out (forward and backward)—with intention and precision, and in harmony with how you're feeling. You're creating your own personal energy mandala, your own Vitruvian Sphere, on top of a perfect foundation, the circular shape of your rebounder. As you move, the energy of the patterns you create can be thought of as speaking to each other, inspiring each other, and waking up the subtle mechanisms in your brain and body that blossom into ever freer and uninhibited motion and feelings of flow.

"Filling in" your Vitruvian Sphere—moving through and tracing in the geometric patterns that your body makes as it flows in and out of different shapes and patterns—takes time. In fact, you can never fill it in completely. Instead, your movements are creating an increasingly complex living mandala that your energy aura inhabits and that evolves and enlivens your physical body. As you work your way through the space around you—as you develop and fill in your Vitruvian Sphere—you can through physical and physiological problems, as well as psychological and energetic blockages.

As all the energy catalyzed by bouncing flows through you, it electrifies the information highways of your muscles, your tripartite brain, your nerves, your veins, your lymphatic system, your bones, and more. Then, something can happen—something very special—as you reach a place where your inspiration and embodied physicality can begin to collaborate as they never have—and perhaps never could have—before.

Suppose you move your left wrist in a way you've never moved it before. This action causes new information to cascade down the channels of your physical system, and a channel that's been blocked for years can open up. Now you've got blood and healing energy moving through the formerly blocked floodgates, and that part of you—and the other parts that are directly connected to it—can begin to heal and work more optimally according to their original designs.

Imagine the Colorado River. The massive flow of water, its intensity, its speed, its sheer volume—taken together, this all created and shaped the Grand Canyon. Yes, it took a long time, but that colossal body of water started out as some melted snow trickling down from the mountains, finding cracks and crevices to flow through. Gradually those fissures became larger and larger fractures, allowing for more water to collect and join forces. The more water that's allowed to collect, the more H_2O molecules work on those rocks and the faster that fracture becomes completely cleared away. Before you know it, a once-restricted pathway is now free and clear. Similarly, old obstructions can be cleared away from your body, just like the rocks that stood in the way of the flowing river.

Yes, this will, of course, take some time. Building your multidimensional personal energy mandala, finding the unexplored spaces of your Vitruvian Sphere, clearing out the obstacles in your physical and energy body—these are all organic processes that must necessarily develop and evolve over time. Note, however, that time itself *is* the fourth dimension, and this is how movement in 4D can be understood. Time is always an element in our movements. For example, it takes between several seconds and several minutes to complete a set of rebounding movements, depending on what exactly you're doing and how fast you're performing them.

We're *already* always part of the fourth dimension: our body participates in its very essence by never being able to completely freeze (other than when we die, and even then it keeps changing). Our conscious mind can go silent, but our body never can—and never does—stop. Our blood pumps, our heart beats, our lungs breathe, and certainly our incredibly numerous and complex cellular processes are ongoing. Our body naturally and elementally participates in the fourth dimension. Becoming aware of time in this way—learning to consciously and lovingly harness it for our own benefit—is the goal here.

As for how our bodies move in and through time, generally time itself seems very directional, as do most things having to do with time that we can observe with our normal perceptions. As far as we're concerned, time always goes forward, never backward. This forward movement of time's arrow seems unstoppable by any conventional means human minds have yet been able to come up with. Einstein's theory of relativity may show that time has no direction in and of itself, and that it's only our perception of time that creates our impression that things must have a beginning and an end—but it sure doesn't feel that way living day to day, year after year. Nope, we seem stuck in time, moving forever forward toward our own ultimate decay and demise.

So what can be done? Time machines and wormhole transporters are technologies still too far away to be worth getting excited about, and these faraway future ideas will in any case do nothing for those crows' feet branching out ever further on the edges of our eyes. But perhaps looking toward future scientific breakthroughs is reaching a little too far away from home anyway. Perhaps there is something that is right in front of us—maybe even right *inside* of us—that can provide us with an effective solution.

Telomeres and Time's Arrow

Can we influence our own personal time's arrow through conscious deployment of our bodies? A *telomere* is a region of repetitive DNA at the end of a chromosome (the structure that carries our genes) and serves as a kind of end cap (like the plastic end cap on shoelaces). Every time a cell divides, the telomere shortens. It keeps on shortening until there's no more telomere left, and then the cell dies. Such cell death directly brings about aging on a cellular level and thus negatively influences lifespan. Put differently, the length of its telomere determines how long a cell can live. Generally speaking,[31] longer telomeres means longer-living cells, which translates to a longer-lived you.

---

31   Some research has shown that in certain cases having *longer* telomeres can be associated with a particular type of lung cancer. See http://www.eurekalert.org/pub_releases/2015-07/uocm-ltl072415.php. The relationship between telomere length, longevity, and cancer risk is not yet understood, but it seems probable that the real key here is the length of your telomeres at a given time compared to their original length, and that having short telomeres does lead to premature cell dysfunction and ultimately cell death.

At first blush, this may sound like a predetermined system. Your chromosome's telomeres are just so long, and that's all you get, right? Time's arrow strikes again? Well, maybe not this time. Your telomeres, science increasingly finds, respond to your lifestyle and your habits, and can be influenced by both exercise and meditation. The implications of this are pretty mind-boggling. By exercising, it seems, you can reverse at least some of aging's effects and *live a longer and healthier life*.

Some of the research shows that *by exercising, you directly act upon your cells to lengthen your telomeres*, thereby giving your cells more time to healthfully divide and conserve the precious genetic material housed within. Also, longer telomeres mean less illness and chronic disease, since your genes will be able to continue to properly express themselves and build and rebuild all your essential components and systems. All of this sounds almost like a real-life time machine—but instead of being something that you step into, it's microscopic and already lives within us, in our very own cells!

A study done in England on 2,400 twins was the first to show promising results as to exercise and telomere length. Questionnaires were given to twins that collected information on physical activity and a few other factors. The results were pretty amazing:

> People who did a moderate amount of exercise—about 100 minutes a week of activity such as tennis, swimming or running—had telomeres that on average looked like those of someone about five or six years younger than those who did the least—about 16 minutes a week. Those who did the most—doing about three hours a week of moderate to vigorous activity—had telomeres that appeared to be about nine years younger than those who did the least. As the amount of exercise increased, the telomere length increased.[32]

One of the many things that we regularly hear from people who have committed to a regular rebounding practice is how their skin feels firmer all over their body, their eyes shine brighter, and they have more energy. Could

---

32   See http://www.edinformatics.com/news/exercise_and_aging.htm.

these results, at least in part, be the physical "side effects" of lengthening telomeres? It certainly seems possible.

Research increasingly indicates that simple lifestyle changes can help reverse the aging process. Our internal clock *can* be turned back. Time's arrow can be reversed. We are not powerless slaves to our genes and our cells. In fact, we can impact them in a real and measurable way.

Fortunately, we don't have to wait around until someone figures out all the intricacies of what does and doesn't affect our telomeres and aging overall. The future of anti-aging technology—at least one element of it—is already right here, right now. We already know for a fact that, on average, exercise lengthens our lives and reduces the risk of illness and chronic disease. A rebound exercise practice is exactly the kind of lifestyle change that helps those telomeres stay long. Rebounding is movement in four dimensions, where you move forward through time, breaking down the blockages in your body and spirit that kept you confined, as well as backward through time, physically making yourself younger the longer and more consistently you engage in the Bounce.

Now it's time to get on your bouncer and *feel* it. Feel the Vitruvian Sphere around you. Let the energy of the sphere tickle your skin. Close your eyes and breathe in the energy aura that surrounds you as you move your arms, fingers, feet, and hips. See with your mind's eye how each movement creates a petal in an ever-evolving mandala that fills your Vitruvian Sphere with unique and complex patterns, as individual to you as your own fingerprints.

Engage with the g-force as your body moves up and down on the rebounder. Spend as long as you can in the moment of weightlessness at the top of the bounce, where you can almost feel wings begin to sprout from your back and lift you away. Touch time with your awareness and experience your movements in a normal trajectory. Then feel how each moment forward is actually a subtle movement back, just like when a wave crashes to the shore and the water is pulled back into the ocean. This is the beginning of what "being bounced" feels like.

"Being bounced" is another way of saying "being in the flow," and that is something we've all experienced at one time or another in our lives, probably all too infrequently. Rebounding is a remarkable way to harness that energy and lift off into the higher dimensions of your own capacities and capabilities. It's in you, around you, above you, below you, and throughout you. You become the Bounce, and soon, with a little extra effort, you will begin to bring that flow into the rest of your life as well.

Chapter 7:

Joy's Journal (the Sequel), the Challenge, and Some Q&As

[These further entries are Joy's personal notes on what it was like—fairly early on in her experience of the Bounce—to take on the substantial challenge Jordan presented to her. While it wasn't always easy, in the end it was more than worth it. Joy gained a bigger, broader, and more definitive understanding of the Bounce's benefits, as well as a visceral experience of the utility of visualizing and working within the Vitruvian Sphere.]

Joy's Journal: The Sequel ("Brave Enough to Try")

It's been almost two months to the day since I first stepped onto my rebounder. Jordan seems quite pleased with my progress so far. And now he thinks I'm probably ready to shoot for a new rebounding milestone.

He's been telling me about a challenge he set for himself in the early days as an experiment—he bounced for 45 minutes every day, continuing for 45 days in a row. He also told me that this personal "marathon" was a huge turning point in his own rebounding experience, because he made an important discovery toward the final stretch of his 45-day marathon. He described it as a different inner state, completely aside from the fitness and aerobic results: he felt a deeper mind-body connection occur, and said it was both fascinating and beneficial to experience.

But describing it in words, Jordan also said, just wasn't possible and wouldn't do me any good. The only way for me to fully experience and understand this enhanced flow state was to get there myself through sheer persistence and determination.

Jordan is really curious as to whether I'll experience a similar state if I go ahead and undertake the same experiment. So of course, he asks if I'm willing to consider making the same 45-day, 45-minutes-per-day commitment.

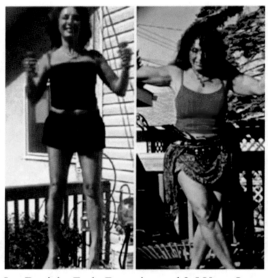

Naturally, I find this very intriguing, and I always like a good challenge, but I also feel some trepidation about whether I'll be able to keep my promise and meet such a

Joy Daniels: Early Bouncing and 2.5 Years Later

goal. I've never bounced nonstop longer than half an hour. By the end of that half hour, I'm already tired. And I can only last that half hour because of my clever choice of motivating songs.

Jordan's challenge calls for continuous bouncing. No sinking down onto the mat for meditative rest breaks. Forty-five minutes is a long time. Really long. And 45 days in a row is a lot—a serious commitment.

My answer? Yes. I'll attempt 45 nonstop minutes of bouncing 45 days in a row. I don't know if I'll make it all 45 minutes for all 45 days. But I'm willing to try.

After all, runners experience a "runner's high" as they "break through the wall" of their previous limits of endurance. It's a well-known result of nearly any kind of extreme "push" accomplished during physical exercise. I had comparable experiences in my dancing days, when I was much younger and able to endure the continuous up-and-down contact with hardwood floors for long periods of time.

So I wonder if I'll experience some kind of a "bouncer's high." Maybe that's what the flow state associated with marathon bouncing is all about—a deep spiritual flow state that goes far beyond the physical. Well, just like he said, the only way to find out is to try it for myself. We'll see!

Filling In My Personal Vitruvian Bubble

I was already familiar with a famous drawing by Leonardo da Vinci. Called the Vitruvian Man, it's a classic image of the human form at its strongest, most beautiful, and best, with multiple limbs superimposed over the outside of a circle.

Jordan refers to his own idea of a "Vitruvian Sphere" or "Vitruvian Bubble," sketching out a conceptual visual of a bouncing person moving through the entirety of the spherical space that surrounds their body.

He says to consciously feel this Vitruvian Bubble surrounding the outer edges of my physical body mass as I rise up into the air and then sink down into the suspended rebounder mat with each cycle of bouncing. He suggests I think of it as an invisible circle of charged air and space surrounding my body, exactly the area covered by my extended legs and arms (or perhaps just a bit longer) as they stretch out into the air. So much like da Vinci's drawing! (Did the secretive master inventor Leonardo invent the rebounder, and not tell anyone?)

Placing attention on the space that I fill and move through during the Bounce, I rapidly feel both lighter and larger—at the same time. I like noticing the difference in how bouncing feels, back and forth between being kind of extra grounded with hand weights, and flying free and light without them. With two months of daily Bounce practice, my physical stamina is much greater, and I've been able to notice that my real-time awareness of my body moving has reached a whole other level.

I'm no longer distracted by tiredness, no longer wondering if I can keep up the pace. Instead, I now consciously *feel* the Bounce. And it feels wonderful, strong, focused, and smooth. There are moments—often toward the final 10 minutes of these long Bounce sessions—that I feel I'm something more than an ordinary human being flying up and down in the air. I've become one with the movement. The Bounce is moving me, rather than my body moving by conscious choice.

I become the Bounce, fully and completely. This must be what Jordan meant by a newly expanded sense of flow. This quote from Fleetwood Mac's song "Rhiannon": "All your life you've never seen a woman taken by the wind." As I discover the inner flow of the Bounce, it feels like I've been taken by the Wind.

Throwing Away the Troubles of a Miserable Day

I had insomnia last night, and then a long, tiring, crappy workday. All day long I was exhausted—physically and emotionally drained—with a tired body and sagging spirit. When I got home I immediately got on my rebounder, wondering whether today, of all days, I could last my full 45 minutes.

As soon as I started bouncing to the music of the Black Eyed Peas, my mood lightened. Instead of further tiring out, I found myself feeling better and better. I felt the day's stress and weariness melting away.

On days like this, arm circles are super energizing for me. The more I do them, the better it feels. Fifty in a row sounds like a lot, but it feels like I could easily just keep on going. And of course, as Jordan *always* points out, if you do an exercise one way (for example, clockwise), then you need to do the opposite way so everything stays properly balanced.

I've invented a fun new variation of arm circles for myself. As my arms circle under, I cross them with closed fists across the center of my chest. Then on the upward bounce I fling my arms upward and outward with hands wide open, fingers splayed, vigorously pushing all my angst outward in a rush. All the troubles of my day leave through my flashing fingers. Whoosh! That feels wonderful.

The Vitruvian Bubble that Jordan taught me to imagine surrounding my body is starting to feel increasingly real and solid. I feel much like a magician casting spells. There's a distinct feeling of power being unleashed as I blast the negativity from my moving fingers while suspended in midair. That is, I can literally shake off all of the "bad stuff" and push it outside of my personal Vitruvian Bubble space—and then it can't get back in.

The next time I'm tempted to skip my daily 45 minutes, I just have to remind myself to get on my rebounder regardless, and watch some of Jordan's very entertaining bounce videos. I almost always immediately feel better and more energized when I do this. It's so fun to watch him. While he does arm circles, one side of his brain keeps up the count, while another keeps up his conversation about how to do it. Bouncing is so perfect for using all of the different parts of one's brain at the same time! Once a process like this is learned by feel, it forever becomes part of your repertoire, simple and easy to do.

I like teaching my body to do things in a newly coordinated way. It reminds me of trying to accomplish that childhood trick of patting your head at the same time you rub your tummy in a circular motion.

Something worth emphasizing is that the music I choose to bounce to is incredibly important for me. We all experience the mood-enhancing effects of listening to our favorite songs and music. Somehow, this effect is magnified when you are bouncing to your own favorite songs. Even completely unfamiliar music resonates on a deeper level. My body becomes an instrument—a part of the orchestra or band—as I add in my own physical and emotional notes through my Bounce.

The Lazy Bounce as Hangover Cure

Speaking of music, last night was Friday, a perfect night for me to host a party. My home was full of musicians jamming together. The evening included lots of good wine, and we stayed up *way* too late. Super fun that night, of course, but then comes the day after.

So right now I feel like total crap. But even in this completely uninspired state, I'm still going to get myself up on my rebounder. I turn on Jordan's bouncing lesson video and follow along as best I can. I take it easy, but keep on going. I figure that as long as I'm still moving and don't get off my rebounder, I'm still with the program, that much closer to hitting my 45 X 45.

Today's restful bouncing is perfect for me. I've discovered, as a big bonus, that gentle, careful bouncing mitigates the ill effects of a well-deserved hangover. This must be due to all that lymph moving around my insides, helping to clear out toxins.

So, today I proved to myself that I really am committed to not missing even a single day of my 45 days in a row.

Eleven Days into the Challenge, I Move from 2D to 3D

This is the 11th day of my 45 X 45 Bouncing Marathon, and I'm in a marvelously happy frame of mind. I can really feel my brain and my body becoming more connected.

Jordan taught me a finger-tapping exercise to do while bouncing. When I first tried tapping my individual fingers on the thumb of the same hand in sequence, my right hand (the hand I write with) was much more coordinated at this than my left hand. But by now, both of my hands are equal. This is a noticeable, fascinating, and unexpected improvement in my coordination.

As I'm bouncing, I now consciously feel my body moving through time as it also moves through space. Here's a metaphor I dreamed up. Imagine what it's like to be a sequence of video images on a flat-screen TV image. You feel quite real, you move, you interact with the things surrounding you—all within that flat screen. Now imagine being that same sequence of video images, but upgraded: this time you're shown on a huge theatrical cinema screen that comes right out at the audience with a vivid 3D perspective. You're the same sequence of video images in either case, but there's just no question that you're so much more impressive and immersively real in 3D.

"Consistently carrying your physical mass in a persistent pattern" is one way Jordan describes filling in the Vitruvian Bubble. Bouncing helps me feel like I accomplish just that in three dimensions. And consciously doing this consistently gives me a feeling of being a strong, steady, and complete physical body, one that knows how to move in a very 3D way. It feels so good, it's hard to express!

Day by day, I find that something about my 45 X 45 bouncing marathon is causing me to notice distinct perceptual changes. This is a new experience for me. More than a physical feeling, it's coming from *inside* me yet radiating outward during my bouncing. By consistently doing the full 45 minutes and passing through a physical endurance "wall," I'm somehow now also passing through a metaphysical wall.

Energy Arc to Add Some Spark to Your Bounce!

My career has been difficult to navigate recently. I've often found myself being a tired, stressed-out girl by the time I come home from work after a long week, and that includes today.

So, naturally, once again it's up on my rebounder I go.

And once again, by the third song I can literally feel new energy flooding through me. I'm just doing simple jumping jacks, up and down, with light weights in my hands, then moving on to arm circles.

Energy Arcing is another concept Jordan suggested, a fascinating inner experience that's fostered by the imagination. It happened the first time for me today.

When my arms reach the top, above my head, there is a momentary inner feeling of electricity, a wee "snap, crackle, pop." I can feel it, and very nearly hear it. And each repetition of the move feels better and better.

With weights in my hands, I've always noticed how "heavy" I feel compared to bouncing light and "free" with empty hands. This makes sense, and is pretty obvious, I suppose. But today, concentrating on the Energy Arcing effect and how I'm actually personally creating it, my whole body feels noticeably lighter and stronger, even with weights.

The weights no longer feel heavy at all. I feel my feet rising higher and faster and lighter off the rebounder mat with each bounce. The weights seem to push me up just as much as they draw me down. Then back up again higher and stronger. It's so much fun to feel both the direct combination of gravity's pull and this uplifting energetic force.

The Fuzzbusting Bonus

Now I understand why this 45 X 45 extended Bounce session marathon is, pardon the pun, a whole jump up from my first casual mini-bounces. It's making me ever more aware of my mind-body connection. The longer I continuously bounce, the more aware I become.

I tried to fit in a nice late-afternoon nap today. Circumstances forced me to wake up earlier than I wanted to. With naps, as you know, either too long or too short leaves you waking up feeling worse than before you nodded off. Right now, I feel all groggy and logy, with my brain all full of fuzz, so to speak.[33]

Despite feeling fuzzy, I do some bouncing. Within the first minutes, I feel my brain rapidly clearing. Whoosh! Whoosh! Whoosh! After 10 minutes, I feel alert and wonderful. All that mind fuzz is simply gone. Seems that when you get your lymph flowing, it clears out the fuzziness from your brain

---

33   We highly recommend watching the "Fuzz Speech" video by Gil Hedley, which you can find at https://www.youtube.com/watch?v=_FtSP-tkSug. It's all about stretching and fascia, and why it's so very important to break up the "fuzz" in your body (which you're given a close look at!).

as well. (And, in fact, I learned from Jordan that in just the past few years a lymph channel that goes directly into the brain was finally discovered, surprising experts in anatomy everywhere.)

The Flow State

Jordan was right. I've begun to experience that wonderful flow state that occurs during long Bounce practices. It moves beyond the simple happy feelings that bouncing creates during shorter sessions. I've been giving a lot of thought to what this flow state is, and how I can put this inner feeling into words.

The more I experience the obvious physical benefits of a Bounce practice, the more connected I also become with the inner workings of the spiritual, mental, and emotional parts of who I am. The more I welcome these inner sensations with conscious intention, the better my body works.

I now feel connected on levels that I never did before. I picture my body as filled with Inner Universes. The cells that create my physical self are constantly interacting, growing, and changing as they literally provide the very basis of my life and health. This is how each of us becomes a human, right from that first moment of conception, before we're even born. Are the trillions of cells that make me who I am aware that they exist? That's another one of the great mysteries of life. To me, it feels like they have a level of awareness, as do all living things. These cells form my Inner Universes, or Inner-Verse.

And then, outside the edge of my skin, there is the great big Outer Universe that we all inhabit. The Outer Universe, or Outer-Verse, is flowing from the external envelope of the space my body inhabits outward toward infinity, with a whole lot of stars and galaxies along the way.

As I'm bouncing, my Inner-Verse and the Outer-Verse connect to become the complete Universe, the Omni-Verse. And what I feel moving through me as I'm bouncing is the Cosmic Flow that connects the two together.

Moving consciously into such flow states while I'm bouncing connects me with this entire process in a way that thoroughly resonates with my experience of being human. I have felt this kind of blissful connection through yoga, for example. And I've experienced similar mind spaces through meditation. And yet, for me, the combination of actively moving through space on my bouncer while experiencing such a flow state is beyond anything I've felt before. Even better, this simply wonderful experience is one I can reliably re-create over and over again, all within the circle of my rebounder.

How does this happen? Is it the airborne antigravity effect inherent in rebounding? Is it more apparent to me now because I set my intention to experience such a thing? Regardless, it's simply so very wonderful to feel this experience of deep connection. And it's all made possible through the use of such a relatively simple device: a descendant of the trampoline, a rebounder. Who would ever have anticipated such a thing?

I still love my little morning mini-bounces. I still value the near-instant stress relief of a short bounce right after a tough day at work, or in the midst of a tough time at home.

But the very best experiences I've had while bouncing consist of nice long times powered by an inspiring choice of alternating fast and slow music. What began as a Bounce Marathon Challenge is now my preferred method of rebounding. As often as my daily life lets me devote a full hour to rebounding, I now do so. Once the multi-level flow state is experienced, it becomes easier to slip into it consciously, almost at will.

My initial months of rebounding rewarded me with well-achieved aerobic and fitness benefits. Now my fitter self allows me to easily complete this 45-day Bounce Marathon Challenge of a daily 45-minute Bounce. And to think of all those many years I thought I'd never be a person who wanted to exercise!

Health Challenges and Opportunities—Q&A

Since launching our Facebook SuperBound® page a few years ago, we've used that platform to help many people start their own practice of the Bounce. In the process, many questions have arisen relating to health challenges and opportunities. This section presents Joy's responses to just a few of those questions in Q&A format.

‖ *What if I'm hurt or recovering from substantial bodily injuries?*

Many people who consider rebounding—including those with injuries, lower back problems, or just the desire to get in shape—wonder if it will be able to work for them.

Q1: Over the past two years I've broken my ankle, torn my ACL and MCL, and fractured my kneecap. Then I incurred a star fracture on the same kneecap a year later. So I'm a little out of shape and strength for sure. I think rebounding will be a great way to get my muscles built back up without injury. I bought an inexpensive rebounder. We'll see how this goes. It's all I can afford right now and I really wanted to get something, so that's what it is, a start.

Q2: Help! I need to lose weight and don't know how....Bloody medication has ballooned me by adding two and a half stone. I am in pain with back problems, so most exercise is out, and I cannot walk far due to breathing problems and pain. Any ideas would be greatly appreciated.

Q3: Joy, I've been watching you rebound now for many months. I would love to get one of these, but how is it on the knees and lower back? I used to work out with weights and belonged to gyms, and even had a trainer—but I still put my back out for six months. So while I am always hesitant to go forward, I so need to tone up and get in shape. What do you recommend?

A: Rebounding is among the lowest-impact, easiest-on-the-body exercises in existence (along with swimming), especially for folks with knee and back challenges. Always check with your doctor first, just to be sure this kind of exercise is okay. As described in chapter 4, I had severe back injuries and problems and was afraid I might never be able to dance again.

However, in all the years since I began regular bouncing, my back and knees have strengthened remarkably, and overall, my regular Bounce practice has proven to be remarkably effective physical therapy for me. In fact, I hate to imagine how I'd feel if I weren't so dedicated to rebounding. I know that when I'm away from my daily Bounce practice when I travel, my pain and symptoms can reoccur. Classic back relief exercises do help, but nothing—absolutely nothing—works as well for me as bouncing.

Just keep in mind that you need to **start very slow and gently**. Begin with simply standing on your rebounder mat and moving back and forth with conscious care. If you feel any discomfort anywhere in your body, shift your weight gently in different directions until you find the "sweet spot" where you can move without pain. Over time, you should find that those uncomfortable areas gain mobility, flexibility, and strength.

We cannot emphasize enough just how important it is **to go slowly**. Work on the rebounder no more than five minutes at a time to begin with in one session. Then rest. You can do this multiple times in a day. And always pay conscious attention to how any injury-sensitive or frequently uncomfortable parts of your body feel.

Your careful patience should be well rewarded by your experiencing a nice, steady injury-free buildup of strength and whole-body functionality.

For ladies only—minding your pees and queues

The question of whether bouncing on a rebounder will lead to sudden, surprising, and possibly very embarrassing need to urinate is one that gets asked a lot! Here are four versions of that same question:

Q1: "Hi Joy. I'm thinking of a rebounder. But I have a weak bladder. In your opinion and experience, would you say I would be able to bounce? Have you heard of people with these issues having any luck with bouncing?"

Q2: "Doesn't rebounding affect the bladder while bouncing? I know ladies have problems sometimes...with the pelvic floor...bladder, etc."

Q3: "After having babies my pelvic floor muscles have never really been as strong. I wonder if all that bouncing up and down on a rebounder will make it better or worse?"

Q4: "I'm not shy about saying I need to strengthen my lower lady muscles, if you get my drift. I sometimes pee a bit just from laughing too hard! Will rebounding help?"

A: This is a question my women friends ask me a lot! Having had two children and a rather weak bladder my whole life, regular rebounding has been remarkably effective as a way to improve and strengthen my core and bladder muscles. Other women who bounce report the same results. No more inadvertent peeing when you cough or laugh. Sure, at first—given the effect of gravity while bouncing up and down—you may feel the need to go pee (just that little bit) within the first couple of minutes. So...you just safely get off the rebounder, go pee (even if just that little bit), and then continue on. While bouncing you can strengthen your core effectively with Kegel exercises. These are basically very easy: you consciously tighten the area (like a small internal flex in), then relax, then flex in, then relax, and so on. The awesome thing about doing this while you are rebounding is that the inner exercise is both extra effective and you can feel it more consciously. After some time of practicing this you will be surprised by how much tighter you are and how much the "need to pee" trigger will lessen even in regular life. You can think of it as being one of the BEST (Bladder Endurance Strength Training) side effects of the Bounce.

Will bouncing likely help depression?

Q: "I have battled clinical depression since I was a teenager. My mind sometimes races with unhappy thoughts; medication has helped, but not always. And the meds have caused weight gain that I've done nothing about, which also makes me depressed. I see how happy you look in your rebounding videos. Do you think rebounding might help?"

A: I really do understand how difficult it is to navigate a path through depression. For me, personally, rebounding has been *an amazing aid to remembering what it feels like to feel happy.* My Bounce practice accomplishes this for me. I have become accustomed to visualizing the circle of my rebounder mat as the place where I "turn off" the outer world at will, and "go inside" for a while. That replenishing and revitalizing mind-space—which some call "Center"—is something each of us carries within. My Bounce practice makes it easy for me to access it. Julia von Flotow, a friend of ours and a gifted life coach, describes the need for all people (whether depressed or not) to access this space:

> *Morning insight:* Having inner quiet can happen anywhere and anytime—it's something you can cultivate through practice. Having a regular daily ritual and committing to reflective practice in a quiet, sacred inner space you create for this purpose can enhance and accelerate your inner growth.

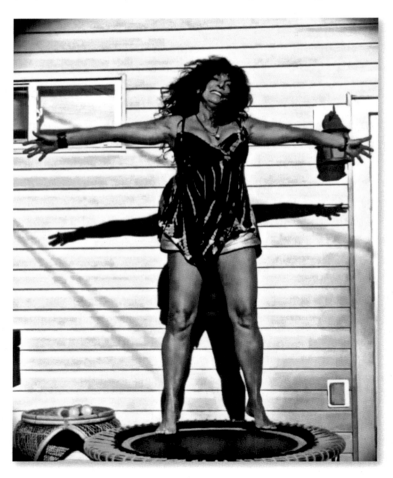

Chapter 8:

Advanced Protocols,
the Limits of Knowledge

[Like the book now known as The Bounce, *Jordan considers himself a work in progress. In this chapter he shares his reflections on the limits of knowledge (especially his own), some new ideas on why bouncing with weights seems to be so effective, and the true nature of the "advanced protocol" he uses for his own daily practice of the Bounce.]*

I started bouncing in 1984 after obtaining a cheap spring-based rebounder. It was an awful experience that I gave up after a few weeks. I next bounced in 2002, on a high-end spring-based rebounder (a Cellerciser) that a friend brought over and urged me to try. I was hesitant, so she held my hand as I got on! I absolutely loved it—right away something inside me said, "Yes! I'm going to do this as much as I can, as often as I can!" As soon as my own new rebounder arrived—it was an American-made unit that I now consider medium quality—I started bouncing daily, and I have been doing that ever since.[34]

---

34 I do miss days occasionally, including when I'm traveling and it's not feasible to strap the rebounder onto the roof of my car. Still, a fair estimate would be 97+ percent of the days since I began.

By profession I'm a writer, so it's not surprising that for 16 of those 18 years of daily bouncing and freely sharing my enthusiasm I've been trying to find a way to write something meaningful and useful on the subject. The urge to write a full-fledged book hit me two months after I started bouncing. My wise friend Jeramy Hale said, "You might not really know enough about it yet," and after thinking it through, I decided he was right. So I put off writing anything for *two whole years* (gasp!) while continuing to avidly bounce, explore, and read everything I could.

The book that I then wrote in 2004—*On The Rebound*—was for the most part much too big and unwieldy to be usable. Since then, I've worked with a number of very talented people on rebounding (editors, illustrators, website designers, even a well-known inventor—many people contributed their energy at one point or another), but I was never able to finish and release something I felt really good about.

That this book is now finished was made possible by two things. First and most obviously—so obvious I don't want to forget to distinctly mention it with profound appreciation and gratitude—is my SuperBound partnership with the unbelievably talented, wise, strong, and beautiful Joy Daniels. I'm thrilled both that we persevered and that we're finally making something happen now that will benefit so many.

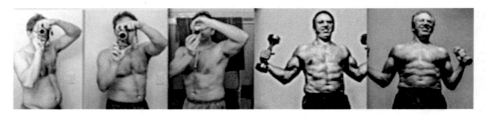

Jordan Gruber, from 2.5 weeks of the Bounce (far left, age 42)
to almost 18 years (age 60)

The Bound(aries) of Knowledge

Second is my realization that (a) since there's a contradiction constantly surrounding how I feel about how much I *actually* know about rebound exercise, (b) I might as well relax, not overthink things, and simply stay curious and open. You see, part of me is *certain* I know more about rebound exercise than ever before. That's true whether I'm instructing friends, offering gentle reframes of questionable or outright false information, or evolving and practicing my own personal brand of the Bounce. But I also now know that, relatively speaking—compared to everything I *could* or *might possibly* know about rebound exercise—I know less than ever. In fact, I often feel like I'm losing ground.

For example, not only do I now know that I do *not* know with certainty the right or best way to bounce, I also know that *there is no one single best or right way to bounce*. The more I see how others bounce, both online and in person, the more I know that each and every human being bounces very differently if left to their own devices and instincts.[35]

Another example: I've come across two ideas in the past year—Doug Brignole's treatise *The Physics of Fitness* (2018, available from http://dougbrignole.com), and the notion of eccentric muscle contractions (what they are, how rebounding seems to automatically make them happen, and what they do for us)—that have opened up new ways of conceptualizing and engaging in my own personal practice of the Bounce.

The finishing of *The Bounce* a month before my 60th birthday comes at the end of the heaviest work phase I've had in many years.[36] So instead of trying to get everything in *The Bounce* perfectly correct, and producing a definitive, comprehensive volume for the ages that captures everything of importance, I decided to trust my instincts and let it all go. I knew that Joy and I would do

---

35   As noted earlier, it's wonderful to bounce along to an online or real-world class if you've got the chance...but you've *also* got to be able to have fun and really get going by yourself and for yourself, both at home and alone, if you're going to make the Bounce a lifelong practice.

36   My other recent book, co-authored with James Fadiman, *Your Symphony of Selves* (Inner Traditions, 2020), is a comprehensive guide to a simple idea. The book's catchphrase is "mental health is being in the right mind at the right time." For me, my selves, personas, or parts include (a) the hardcore writer and editor typing these words to you; (b) the Broadway- and classical music-loving part who had his first-ever voice lessons last year; and (c) the part of me that *loves* to bounce.

William James, the founder of American psychology, wrote about "social selves" in the 1890s! Learning to shift in and out of these different parts of who we are—instead of being triggered or switched into a self that isn't a good fit for the moment—is life-changing. And as soon as you take your own selves or parts seriously, it becomes much easier to do this.

the best we could with a certain set of materials within a certain timeframe. The result is the book you are now reading. May it serve you well.

Connecting Heaven and Earth: Vitruvian Bound By Breath and Gravity

I spontaneously drew the image on the next page on my home office whiteboard (in the same room where I do most of my bouncing) about six months ago. This happened soon after I became familiar with Doug Brignole's previously mentioned book, *The Physics of Fitness* (Healthy Learning Publishing, 2018) Let's start with a brief look at some of Doug's ideas.

A bodybuilding champion and former Mr. California, Doug subtitled his book "The Analysis and Application of Bio-Mechanical Principles in Resistance Exercise." He spells out the book's central thesis and game plan in the introduction's fourth paragraph:

> What is most important to understand is that the human body is essentially a system of pulleys and levers. Muscles are the "pulleys" and our bones (limbs) are the "levers." Thus, the principles of physics (i.e., "classical mechanics"), which apply to all things that are structural and/or mechanical, also apply to the human body. These physical principles, combined with some basic rules regarding the human musculoskeletal system and muscle physiology, allows us to clearly identify which exercises are best for each muscle group.

Doug, then, uses his understanding of classical physics and body physiology to carefully describe which exercises are correctly or incorrectly (most efficiently) using levers (bones/limbs) to leverage muscles (pulleys) being targeted with the ideal motion for that muscle (moving in the right direction, in the right plane, and at the right angle). The takeaway for us is that depending on *exactly* how we hold and move a hand weight (or just our arm), it will make use of and leverage our entire physical system—our bones and limbs (levers) and muscles (pulleys), and from a more holistic perspective all our connective tissue as well—in a very distinct way.

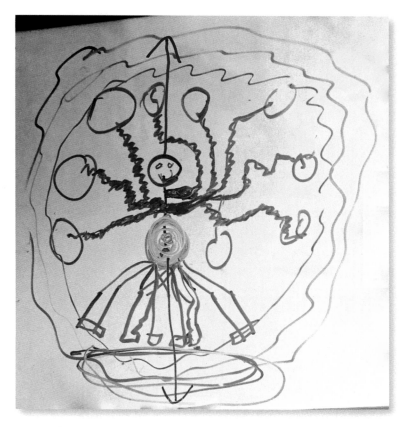

Jordan's Whiteboard Sketch: "One Big Picture of the Bounce"

Most people intuitively understand Doug's idea of leverage: if something is farther away from you, it's going to take more effort to lift it and hold it up. Suppose you have a pair of five-pound handheld weights. If you're holding them at shoulder height, it's intuitively obvious that your arms and shoulders will tire out much more quickly if they are held at arm's length than if they are held in toward your shoulders. In this way, Doug's ideas help explain why the move from two- to three-pound handheld weights requires much, much more strength and energy (and coordination, balance, and breath) if you're using them for highly leveraged activities like arm circles or even simple overhead presses.

Previously what I've said to people is that if you're in the middle of bouncing and you rotate your shoulders in or out just a bit, or raise your arms up or down a little, or change the angle or arc through which you're moving a weight, or change the position of your hips or legs...any of these tiny changes affects your entire system. If you place attention on it, you can feel subtle changes in the amount of energy and strength required to do the same movement. Doug's book, system, and nomenclature clarify a great deal, and suggest many possibilities worthy of further exploration and elaboration.

Another way of thinking about this is to conceive of the body as being a tensegrity structure. R. Buckminster Fuller coined the term "tensegrity" to describe "self-tensioning structures composed of rigid structures and cables, with forces of traction and compression, which form an integrated whole." When you're bouncing, the body can readily be seen or experienced as a tensegrity structure in just this sense.

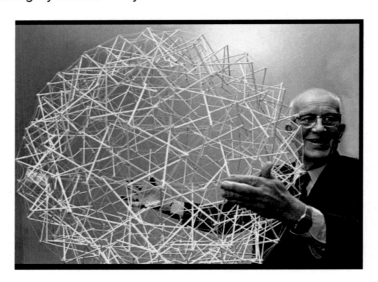

R. Buckminster Fuller with tensegrity structure

In my earlier whiteboard sketch, what pass for arms (with circles at the end as hands) show breaks in three places to indicate that these breaks or leverage nexuses occur at the shoulder, elbow, and wrist. Depending on which of these joints are in play and depending on exactly how you're moving a weight—exactly in what direction, at what angle or arc, with how much force and weight—you can substantially and even radically change the total forces in play that your system is required to produce and adapt to.

I wrote Doug to ask him about applying his ideas to rebound exercise. He was very kind, but not all that fond of "ballistic" exercise, and cautioned me that exercising on a trampoline as I described it could easily overload muscles and potentially be dangerous.

And that's *exactly* why Joy and I recommend using such low-poundage handheld weights, especially at first. But let's take a step back. Conceptually, you can use a rebounder for:

- Diagnostic and exploratory purposes
- Strengthening purposes
- Rehabilitation purposes

Given that you can so effectively leverage the body while bouncing, it becomes very easy—especially when using light (and, cautiously, medium) handheld weights—to diagnose or surface any problems. Going just a bit further, you can also explore the limits of what you're safely capable of. For example, when I move up from three- to four-pound D-shaped dumbbells, not only am I using weights that seem at least twice as heavy (even though they're really only a third heavier), but many more "places"—for example, ways of holding my body and limbs, arcs and vectors of movement, and the outer edges or what I can reach and how far I can extend myself within my personal Vitruvian Sphere—become difficult or impossible to smoothly reach or easily flow into and out of.

Although I've only increased the weight by a single pound, the leveraged tensegrity nature of bouncing very quickly brings me to—and allows me to explore—my own personal limits. This can be a very thorough diagnostic and exploratory process, because it happens in both a 3D way—since we're actively moving in three dimensions on a bouncer—and in a 4D way, that is, over time, as movements are repeated many times in a single session over some duration of time. Once we've diagnosed or explored our limits, we can consciously move to strengthen and rehabilitate the muscles and connective tissue involved—especially if we work closely with our breath and stay conscious and conservative about any "bad" pain that we might feel. (Again, if you have any question whatsoever about pain, just stop.)

What about the rest of my sketch? Doug Brignole has helped us see how to break down the movements we do on a rebounder—and the forces required—into their individual scientific components. In this sense, we can conceptualize separate muscles, limbs, joints, etc., and say exactly what is going on with each one of them depending on what we're doing. But at the same time, it's crucial to remember that ultimately the human body is really just *one* thing. Your body is a single integrated whole, and the intention or will-force that motivates that whole single body—that initiates action and movement—is located in the center of the abdomen, just below the navel, and sometimes called the *hara* or *tantien* by certain Eastern traditions and martial arts.

When I drew that image, I conceptualized the hara—very roughly indicated as an orange circle below the arms and above the legs—as being where movement actually originates when we're bouncing. This brings us back to the notion of pushing down and through our core muscles to first get motion started on a bouncer. So at the same time that we can see ourselves technically through the "physics of fitness" lens, we can also holistically and energetically see ourselves as a single entity whose motion is generated somewhere in the center of our beings (which is also roughly where our center of mass is).

And how is that source of will and motion energized, coordinated, and brought into use? Through breath. Breath initiates and synchronizes our movements, as our bodies are handling forces and being leveraged in many different ways through the physics of fitness. And at the same time, all of this is happening within our Vitruvian Sphere, the energy egg that we generate and that surrounds us.

Within that sphere, powered by gravity (and our mat–springs/bungee-powered bouncer, roughly indicated under my feet), we move up and down along the image's red arrow as we energetically connect Heaven and Earth. Try thinking of yourself as a living filament, an embodied vessel of life force connecting that which is above and that which is below.

Thought Experiment: Eccentric Contractions and 3D Micro-Failures

That's where my thinking was for quite a few months, until I met Michael Sandler, the co-founder of Inspire Nation. After I described the Bounce to Michael, he said something like, "You might want to consider that eccentric contractions may be playing a big role here in its effectiveness." When I went online, I saw that Michael was right on target.

A "concentric" contraction is a contraction while a muscle is shortening, like what happens with your biceps when you curl a weight toward yourself. But when you then let your arm down while holding that weight, an "eccentric" contraction occurs, that is, a contraction while lengthening, sometimes called a "braking contraction."

A great deal has been written about eccentric contractions, and we're not going to be able to get deeply into it this late in the game. What's most important for our purposes is that eccentric contractions can often be stronger and more powerful than concentric contractions, and they also may build strength more quickly. Assuming this is true—let's just call this whole section a "Gedanken" or thought experiment—consider that when you're bouncing, every time you sink into the mat, you experience eccentric contractions in your quadriceps and hamstrings. That is, your leg muscles are necessarily automatically braking as gravity and the mat slow you down through your descent.

Moreover, as you go through many bounce cycles of rising and falling, depending on how you hold and use your limbs and and especially handheld weights, you will potentially experience a variety of eccentric contractions at different phases of what you're doing. For example— assuming you are healthy, ready, and in an experimental mood—take a pair of two-pound hand weights, laterally raise them to shoulder height at arm's length, and hold them there while you gently bounce up and down, keeping your feet on the mat as your center of mass rises up and down a few inches. Try to experience both the concentric and eccentric contractions in your shoulder muscles as you power your movement mainly through your core and lower body.

Then, if and when you're ready, take this to the next level (ha ha). While continuing to slowly bounce up and down without your feet leaving the mat, raise your arms in an arc overhead as far as is comfortable for you, beginning to come up above your head, but do it very slowly...in several small steps...and then lower them very slowly...again in several small steps.

If you think about it, this means that as you go through multiple bounces while slowly raising and lowering the hand weights like this, during part of that time—when your arms are coming down back to shoulder height— your shoulder muscles are experiencing eccentric contractions. But your legs are going through eccentric contractions at the same exact time. So during roughly half of the bouncing cycle—especially if you see your body as really being "just one thing"—you'll be experiencing a kind of doubly reinforced eccentric contraction throughout your entire body.

All this got me to thinking about the use of light handheld weights and muscle failure. For muscles to get bigger and stronger, they first have to reach "failure"—when they are too fatigued to do any more. (And then you need rest and proper nutrition, including sufficient protein.) Lots of information exists on why and how this happens, and over the past few years, there has been increasing agreement that *failure reached through the use of light weights can be very effective at causing muscle growth*. For example, in 2017 Chris Beardsley wrote, "Over the last few years, researchers have discovered that it is possible to achieve meaningful muscle growth when lifting light weights, so long as sets are performed to muscular failure."[37]

What, then, might be deduced about the potential impact of using the kind of light hand weights I typically recommend (and often use myself) for the Bounce? Suppose you're using light handheld weights for a Vitruvian Sphere practice where you're working to fill in, occupy, and move through the entirety of the physical and energetic space that surrounds you. Depending on exactly what you're doing and how you're leveraging your personal tensegrity system, it becomes quite possible to reach a series of what I think of as "micro-failures" as smaller and then larger muscle systems reach fatigue if not failure.

---

37   See https://medium.com/@SandCResearch/what-does-training-to-failure-actually -achieve-2837460c5f0f.

A quick research scan revealed that for maximum muscle activation and growth, the largest muscle complexes and central core of fibers have to be brought into play. So if you're doing seated rows, you have to move a good deal of weight to bring your biggest sets of connected back muscle fibers completely into play and have them fully fire.

This might at first seem like an obstacle to getting to muscle fatigue and failure through bouncing with light handheld weights, because smaller muscles, like those in our arms and wrists, will tire out before we can bring the rest of what's being targeted into play. Suppose you're doing overhead presses while bouncing, and have done 30 or 40 repetitions with three-pound weights. At this point, your wrist, hand, and finger muscles could be getting too tired and fatigued to continue, often long before your shoulders are fully worked, activated, and near failure.

But! All you have to do is rotate your wrists in or out, or change the angle a little, and then you can keep going until the bigger muscle groups and fibers in your shoulders receive the workout they need to reach fatigue and come close to failure, and then repair, grow, and strengthen. (With D-shaped handheld weights, you can put your fingers or wrists through the middle, taking take some or nearly all the load off these extremities.)

The Advanced Bouncing Protocol: Mental Models and the Magic of Intention

Working with a life coach, I decided that on days when I couldn't get to the gym, I'd go ahead and rebound longer at home and do my "advanced weights protocol." The only problem: I didn't have one—an advanced weights protocol—at least not in the sense of a written-down plan I'd consistently and successfully followed.

Not that I hadn't tried. I'd constructed all sorts of plans—sets of bounces I would rigorously and religiously go through, ways I would bounce for certain periods of time, and so on. But when I actually start bouncing on any given day, almost all of this always falls away. So I've come to realize that if I do have an advanced protocol, it's a mental one, a mindset that I bring to the Bounce. My current mental model is based on (a) the above image I drew on my whiteboard, (b) my understanding of the physics of fitness, and (c) my evolving thinking around eccentric contractions and micro-failures.

By this point, I have a pretty well developed mental model. Plus, I use a variety of weights every time I undertake the Bounce to further explore what I know, to see what I can learn, and to further strengthen, explore, and rehabilitate my body, mind, and spirit. I'll frequently come up with a new idea and then test it for weeks in a row, sometimes permanently incorporating it into my practice.

Recently, for example, I realized that for many of the movements I do with light hand weights, it's possible to hold them in my hands *Up*, *In*, *Down*, and *Out*, that is, in four different basic ways or orientations:

- Up (hands up)
- In (hands facing each other)
- Down (hands facing down)
- Out (hands facing out; this is the most difficult position, and not always possible, as it involves rotating out your wrists, forearms, upper arms, and shoulders)

Suppose you are performing multiple repetitions of any given movement or exercise with light handheld weights while you're bouncing. By rotating through all four of these positions—staying with each one for multiple repetitions and then moving to the next—you bring into play many more leveraged configurations of your body and its systems than if you just bounced using just one of these positions. As simple an exercise as bicep curls becomes more interesting, complex, and productive if you go through all four hand positions and do sufficient repetitions to bring the smaller muscles you are using to fatigue or failure in each position before moving on to the next one.

Fortunately, by now I typically don't have to think about any of this. I just know it. I have a fully developed and reliable mental model, so I can just follow my instincts and the music I'm listening to. I pretty much always know what I'm going to do next while I'm bouncing. Maybe not always, but the vast majority of the time.

One last thing I recently discovered this way is that my bouncing sessions are best when I step into what I think of as my "Big Body." This means that while I'm bouncing, usually with weights, I find myself standing up taller—stretching both vertically and horizontally—breathing in and out as fully as possible, essentially willing myself to both loosen up and enter into the most physically expanded and extended version of myself possible.[38] Going through the four positions like this—Up, In, Down, and Out—is even more interesting, intense, and rewarding.

As with so many things, our intention is what's most important. If you hold the intention that bouncing will make you happier, healthier, and stronger—and you put in your time—then this will very likely happen. If you intend to give the Bounce a good try, and you follow the advice in this book, there's a good chance you'll be rebounding for the rest of what will likely be a healthier and longer life than it would otherwise have been.

So ask yourself: "What, really, is my intention?" You see, there's zero doubt that bouncing is highly effective (as well as fun and easy). If your intention is to get healthier and stronger, then most likely that can happen in a pretty straightforward way, as long as you go slow at first and then steadily apply yourself.

The great thing is this: you can easily find out for yourself. And if you happen to not like the Bounce, then you can just stop. But if you *do* like it, your life may end up improving considerably both now and in the long run.

---

38   I see myself as stepping into different movie or book characters as I do this, ones capable of holding that "bigger me" and producing the energy and presence needed to get there. The body may be one thing, but in some ways, as per the healthy multiplicity idea, the mind is many.

Chapter 9:

Conclusion—The Future of Rebound Exercise Is You!

The End of This Book;
The Beginning of Your Own Practice

We've both been bouncing nearly every day for a long time now, and we plan to continue doing so for the rest of our lives. It's super fun, and we've had great (and sometimes truly super) results that have exceeded our initial expectations in many ways.

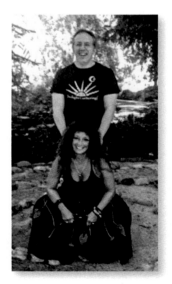

That's what we want for you too. Whatever you're looking to do—lose weight, tone up, build muscle, get sick less, increase your aerobic capacity, improve your balance, be happier—a regular practice of the Bounce may really help. We want you to seriously consider rebound exercise, then try it, and then tell your friends, family, and co-workers. We want you to spread this good news to everyone who wants a stronger immune system. And most of all, we want you to do this for yourself, not just because it's possible, but because you deserve it.

Our vision is for the Bounce to become ten—or a hundred, or a thousand—times more popular than it is now, a premier fitness category that everyone immediately thinks of along with practices like martial arts, weight lifting, and yoga. The SuperBound project is dedicated to making this happen—to enlightening the world about and through rebound exercise—and we strongly feel that if you take what you find in this book and apply it, it will likely dramatically change your life for the better. In fact, we'd like to turn now to some stories and pictures from friends of ours whose lives did in fact improve substantially once they began their own version of the Bounce.

Bouncing Friends from Around the World

Cynthia Stevenson (Sydney, Australia)

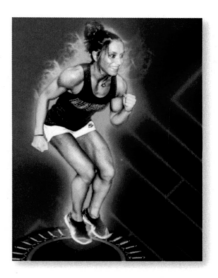

"I can honestly and wholeheartedly say rebounding has changed my life. Having dealt with extremely bad feet all my life, with no arches and having my Achilles on the verge of snapping, I was told by many doctors and podiatrists that my choice of profession (fitness) was a bad one. This was something I was simply not willing to accept. It was through my own research that I stumbled across rebounding and its benefits. It was worth a shot to try strengthening my feet, ankles, and Achilles, as it had gotten to a point where I could not walk down a supermarket aisle without my ankles giving way so I'd collapse in the middle of the fruit and veg section, with people stopping to ask if I was okay!

"I started bouncing regularly in my own time, and within six months my ankles and Achilles were noticeably stronger and no longer giving way on me. It was truly a miracle. I was so happy and excited with the results that in 2011 I started my own group fitness business with my husband, RICO Group Fitness, teaching classes in various locations around Sydney, Australia. We now have a suite of seven different types of classes, with our most popular class being our rebounding class: BOUNCE. The feedback we get from our participants is an overall sense of well-being, increased fitness, and stronger joints. It proved that my results were not just from a placebo. I bounce up to four times a week and give thanks every day to my faithful rebounder, who, again, has not only saved my life but changed it for the absolute better."

Jeramy Hale
(Penn Valley, California, USA)

"I am always looking for effective and easy solutions for movement and well-being, especially ones I don't have to go someplace to do. Can I do it in my home, can I do it in my yard, can I do it on the floor, can I make it simple? The answer with rebounding is a resounding YES!"

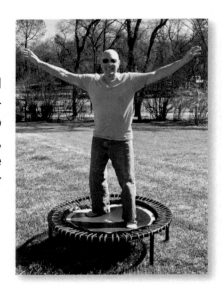

Kelly Angelina Munroe
(Nanaimo, British Columbia, Canada)

"When I first started bouncing, I had a bad rotator cuff and couldn't lift my arm above my shoulder. I started bouncing and it went away. The miracle rebounder, I call that!"

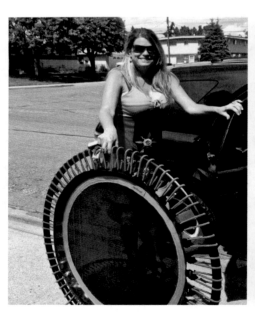

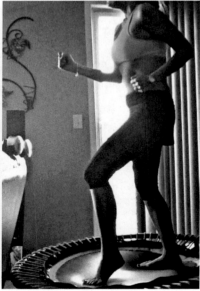

Faye Lewark Daniels
(Statesville, North Carolina, USA)

"I recommend rebounding for anyone with a balance issue. It's the best gift I have given myself."

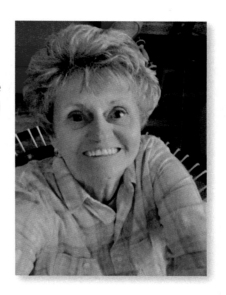

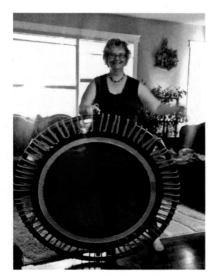

Samantha Rae Jackson
(Calgary, Alberta)

"Bouncing is excellent stress relief. PLUS it is FUN!"

The Winters—The Family That Bounces Together!
(Healdsburg, California, USA)

Phoenix: "The rebounder was one of the only ways I could make myself consistently exercise throughout high school. It's so easy to just put on headphones and see how many songs I can bounce through. It's extra nice when I have something to do on the computer: any time I need a break, I can just get up and exercise for a few minutes."

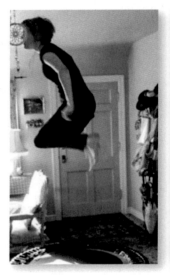
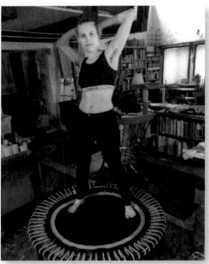
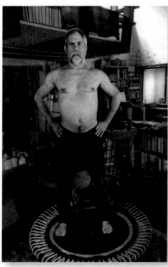
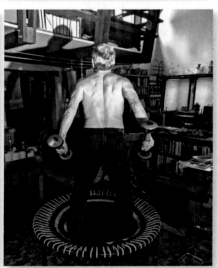

Jeffry: "The rebounder is the ONE exercise regimen I've been able to stick to, on and off, but mostly on, since I got mine about eight years ago. I always go back to it because it feels good to do it and I feel SO much better after. Twice a week is enough to make a huge difference in my life but I like it better when I do four. It's amazing how much of a full body workout it is."

Michelle Robertson
(Wagga Wagga, New South Wales, Australia)

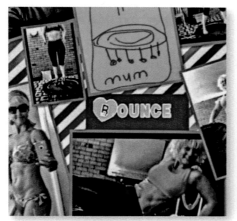 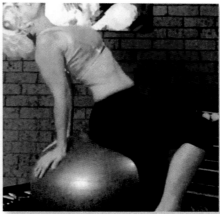

"*The Bounce* is an exciting new book about rebounding and its benefits, and everything else about bouncing that you might be surprised to learn! And my kids are so supportive and proud of me in my love of rebounding."

Twyla Johnson
(Victoria, British Columbia, Canada)

"I remember the day when my rebounder was delivered. It was a beautiful summer day, so I set it up outside. As I took those first bounces, a glorious, familiar feeling of freedom overcame me. It was so reminiscent of my childhood spent on horseback, bounding through the countryside. Pure joy and so good for my soul!"

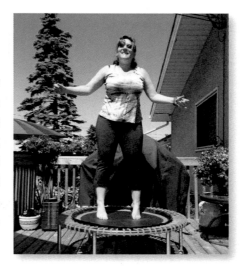

Kathy Scally Abrignani
(Warren, Michigan, USA)

Kathy began the Facebook page 'Rebounding Rocks' in 2014. Her love of rebounding has inspired thousands of people and the fitness and rebounding community she has fostered continues to grow.

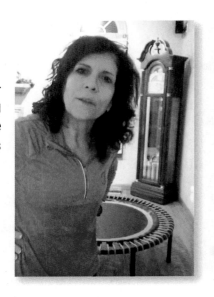

"Rebounding rocks—one of the best joys in life"

Tom McCook
(Moss Beach, California, USA)

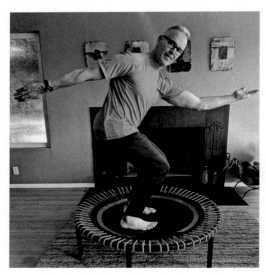

"Rebounding is a perfect tool as part of any health and fitness program. I use mine multiple times a week and feel it has a superb organizing, enlivening and health enhancing effect on each system of the body. I use it for cardio, balance and conditioning and as a quick effective movement break during the work day!"

Karen Ippolito
(Vancouver, British Columbia, Canada)

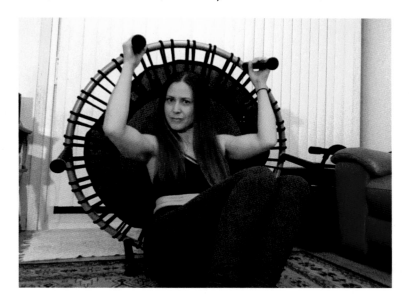

"After putting the children to bed, I found time to rebound while watching the final season of *How I Met Your Mother*. LOVED IT! Easy breezy: low back felt great, and I could relax the tension. Tight IT band and lateral quadriceps were shifted as my core stabilizers were activated, and I felt the energy move from the outer muscles to my center. Kundalini awakened. Root chakra energized. Felt light and free as arms moved effortlessly.

"After 20 minutes of gentle bouncing, I felt energized and clear. The cloud is already lifting, and I am more confident in who I am and what I believe. There was definitely an activation of my core values along with the awakening of my core strength."

More Testimonials from Our Wonderful Friends Who Love the Bounce

Marina C.: "I showed your videos to my four-year-old and I'm getting her a bouncer. We watch your SuperBound bouncing videos before bedtime. She finds it calming."

Debbie D.: "Hey girl, I have finally made a decision...I am going to buy a good rebounder...It's a big investment and I haven't purchased one yet because I made a promise to myself that I wouldn't carelessly spend unless I was sure I was going to use the bouncer. I have had many pieces of equipment over the years that I was excited about when I first got them, and then after the excitement wears off they sit...This includes our hot tub...Because I have held off for so long now and my desire to have a rebounder is just as strong now as it was last year, I figure I will be dedicated to it."

Jeffry W.: "My teenage daughter uses my rebounder often. She has two PE hours each day (at school) and is taking dance. Bouncing is helping her work out the soreness. We gave up our spa membership, so after a few more months our rebounder will be paid for, and it will serve us for decades. It's a GREAT way to exercise. You don't have to go anywhere, so you actually do it. You don't have to dress a particular way or be concerned how you look to other people because you're at home. You can do it five minutes at a time if you want or you can do it (after months of working up to it) for an hour a pop. I'm up to about a half hour on my long bounces and about 15 minutes on the short ones."

Jeremy E.: "When I bounce, it makes me laugh, which is a great way to start any day! In this way it strengthens both my emotional self and my physical well-being."

Twyla J.: "Yesterday I was in a holistic health store and noticed that they now sell bungee cord rebounders. There was a man about 35 years old, tall and fit, bouncing gently up and down on one. His eyes were closed and the look on his face was pure bliss. It instantly transported me back to when I got on my own rebounder for the first time—freedom. Fun. Bliss. Like riding a horse. 'It's fun, isn't it,' I said, and he broke out into a huge grin. 'I want one so bad!' By the way, I told him to check out SuperBound because he was asking me questions when he found out that I had one."

Kelly Q.: "I am going to get a rebounder—awesome! I'm a pretty dedicated person once I start something. Very excited about this. I haven't been this excited about something to do with working out in a long time. The thing is, I don't see it as working out. Bonus!!!!"

Lisa L.: "I went from avoiding exercise completely for a while to bouncing on a rebounder to all of my favorite music. I LOVED IT RIGHT FROM THE START! It gave me so much energy and complete joy! I felt like a little kid again, bouncing on the bed! You can't help but love life when you're bouncing up and down! My legs look awesome and my spirit shines! I'm thinking about how I bounce to my own rhythm. I happen to have grown up in the new wave and punk rock era. I bounce to those tunes. A little faster. A little bit silly and artistically 'creative.' Ha ha! But that's what I enjoy! Sometimes I stop bouncing and GROOVE...then I bounce again! LOL!! I LOVE IT!!"

Amy H.: "Rebounding is FUN. It doesn't feel like work—it feels like flying. I love the weightless sensation and that it is a low-impact but great cardio workout. I love the improved sense of balance too."

Gina P.: "That moment in your life when your young son says, 'Mom, do you know how old Joy is? Have you seen her pictures? She is in GREAT SHAPE!'—and the challenge is on. My sons used to tell me that when I turned 50, I needed to look like that Bowflex® lady that was 50...Now they have turned it up a notch. Challenge accepted! Rebounding, here I come!"

Denise B.: "One of the things I know is that it gets my heart rate up very quickly, which makes me happy that I'm getting good cardio. I always feel lighter spirited after jumping, no matter what mood I was in before I started."

Katrina M.: "Ten years ago I bought a little rebounder. I have been using it ever since. It has saved my physical health. I was a runner when I was young. But my knees gave out and I was so sad because I could no longer walk my dog. I saw the little mini-trampoline and thought, 'Perhaps this might help me strengthen my legs.' And over time it did!!!"

Ginger R.: "My beautiful, gorgeous, fantastic, oh-so-smooth rebounder finally came! I stepped up on what felt like a spongy cloud...and I was in heaven...My first wee jump! Yesterday I jumped three times for three-minute sessions, which didn't seem like much, but I'm taking things slow and working my way up. Yet, to be quite honest, none of that would give me what I'm looking for without a combination of mind, body, and spirit. And I knew when I saw you that you were all about that as well."

Jeramy H.: "I just want to say that in my method, my feet DO leave the mat many times...but just a little, so that it's a very shallow bounce. I like to find a personal balance between the benefits of physical movement and what I refer to as the 'internal arts'...the awareness of—and movement of—energy for health and well-being."

Janice D.: "Bound to revitalize the mind, body, and soul! I love the experience; the 10-minute sessions I strive to work in are very rejuvenating."

Karen M.: "My little girl is four years old. She loves to bounce on our rebounder. Her baby brother watches her and laughs. His turn next!"

Annika H.: "Rebounding has been so good for me. My body says thank you—to myself, and to you, Joy! It wouldn't have happed without you. It's a quite rare exercise form in Sweden still. When I sprained my ankle 3 years ago, the training I did on the rebounder was better than any physiotherapy! I got so much flexibility back that an injury I have had in left ankle, since 12 years of age, healed. My horseback riding teacher was amazed that I had the same flexibility in both feet after 30 years of riding...it was truly wonderful, because symmetry is very important when riding a horse."

Now It's up to You

Our current life and times are both wonderful and filled with abundant challenges. For many, one of the most frustrating things is feeling that so much of what's going on is completely out of our personal control. Politics, climate change, dealing with viral pandemics like COVID-19 (still peaking in the USA as this book is being finished)—taken together, it can all be quite overwhelming.

One thing we *do* have control over is making the best choices for becoming and being as strong, healthy, and emotionally centered and happy as possible. A regular practice of the Bounce accomplishes all of that—which, of course, is why we wrote this book!

As we have written, read, edited, and eventually finalized each of these chapters, we consistently tried to imagine ourselves in your place, reading *The Bounce*, possibly being introduced to rebound exercise for the very first time.

Will you be intrigued by our experiences and entertained by our ups and downs? Will we inspire you to try out rebound exercise for the first time? Or, for those who tried bouncing in the past but never managed to stick with it, will our stories, inspiration, and easy-to-follow instructions motivate you to give the Bounce another try?

We hope you will find many things in this book that speak to you personally. If that's indeed the case, and if rebound exercise makes sense to you—if the Bounce appeals to you on any level (and you have medical clearance)—then please give it a go.

And if you do give it a go, we're thrilled to imagine you making the Bounce an ongoing part of what will no doubt be a longer, more energetic, and healthier life. Good luck, stay safe, have fun, get as fit as you like, and enjoy the heck out of the Bounce!

Appendix A:

A Brief History of Rebound Exercise in America

This isn't the first time rebound exercise has been enthusiastically proposed as the answer for those wanting a fun, new, and effective way to get great exercise (and boost their immune system). The first major rebounding explosion was back in the 1980s, pioneered by Albert ("Al") E. Carter. He is called the "father of rebound exercise" because of his lifelong commitment to rebound exercise, his development and marketing of early rebounders and other rebounding-related products, and his strong focus on education and the connection between rebound exercise and better health.

Carter was an athlete through and through. He received a full wrestling scholarship to the University of Utah and later founded "Gymnastics Fantastics," a professional trampoline troupe that toured and performed in front of half a million people from 1974 to 1975.

He trained his own children to be part of the troupe, and it wasn't long before he noticed some changes in them. Their stamina and fitness had improved dramatically: his daughter could out arm-wrestle any of the boys in her grade at school! Carter also noticed their great degree of both physical coordination and mental alertness, which led him to suppose that something fundamental about rebounding must have initiated these changes. Carter's research resulted in his bestselling first book, *The Miracles of Rebound Exercise*, published in 1977. The updated book, *The New Miracles of Rebound Exercise,* is still in print.

By 1981, interest in rebounding blossomed into a full-blown phenomenon, and the first edition of Harry and Sarah Sneider's *Olympic Trainer: Fitness Excellence through Resistive Rebounding* was published. It seemed like everyone was bouncing onto on the bandwagon (and the nearest rebounder), and more and more manufacturers mobilized to take advantage of the increasing demand.

Unfortunately, this huge spike in interest flooded the market with cheap, poorly made units that broke down quickly. One report said that 1.5 million units were sold in 1983 alone. Offshore companies joined in the frenzy but cut costs so greatly that quality suffered. Plus, the low prices these companies charged for their low-quality equipment contributed to American rebounder companies being driven out of business.

Such low-quality equipment inevitably began to take a physical toll on those actually using it. It really isn't that fun or pleasant—and can be downright dangerous—to bounce on a bad rebounder. By 1985, the initial fad had pretty much faded away.

Al Carter later made an interesting observation: the contrast between rebounding and other, more traditional forms of exercise might have led to some resistance, unrealistic wariness, and outright skepticism by those who had specialized in and dedicated years of training to other forms of exercise. Carter felt that this unconscious resistance to change might have led some of those who should have been natural allies of rebound exercise to instead dismiss it.

But with a number of celebrity endorsements from the likes of Bob Hope, Ronald Reagan, and Jack LaLanne, among others, plus the ongoing availability of a few brands of well-made rebounders, the candle of awareness was kept lit. Moreover, several scientific studies and a few books were published during the rest of the 1980s and early 1990s. In 1987, Harvey and Marilyn Diamond endorsed rebounding in their best-selling *Fit for Life* book, and in 1990 Tony Robbins endorsed rebounding in his book *Unlimited Power*. (Tony, as shown in the 2016 Netflix documentary *I'm Not Your Guru*, likes to revive himself by bouncing in between sessions when he's leading large intensive workshops.) And in 1991, Dr. Morton Walker published *Jumping for Health*.

On the one hand, then, there were decent rebounders available, and the Bounce still had its hard-core devotees. But because of a mass experience of poor equipment and a lack of robust support and know-how, many people simply put their rebounders away in garages, sheds, and basements, where they saw little use and frequently rusted. On the previous page is a picture of Jordan's very own 1984 rebounder with its springs and frame finally rusting away.

Next, martial arts trainer J.B. Berns' book *Urban Rebounding* (2000), and his associated spring-based rebounder and training DVDs, helped evolve the practice of rebound exercise in some important ways. In his own words, "I created the Urban Rebounding workout many years ago because I had a terrible martial arts injury to my right knee and I needed a workout that was easy and gentle on my joints, but at the same time challenging where I could control the intensity level."

Having found this solution to his own health challenges, he built a business that brought the benefits of rebounding to others, and created a program— with both rebounder equipment and a guided exercise plan—that could be used in group fitness classes at gyms, as well as a rebounder packaged with videos that brought those same workouts to the home living room. Berns gained some nationwide publicity and helped reinvigorate rebound exercise and introduce it to many.

Berns' style of fitness workout videos and in-person classes has shown an uptick in recent years. You'll find lots and lots of rebound exercise classes and programs on YouTube—into the thousands or more—and some of the quality vendors, including bellicon, are regularly putting out their own video lessons and classes. (For example, our Australian friend Cynthia Stevenson of RICO Group Fitness, whom you can see in chapter 9, teaches a *very* aerobically intensive class on a spring-based rebounder.)

As a reminder, we're all in favor of watching and following as many online rebounding fitness classes as you like (and we may even offer some of our own), as long as doing so doesn't begin to lead you away from the knowledge that *you don't need anyone or anything else*—except maybe a way to play music—*to safely and intelligently develop, sustain, and thrive with your own practice of the Bounce.*

But probably the most significant development right now is that you can finally get a decent bungee-based rebounder for only two or three hundred dollars. Basically, following the bellicon company's revolutionary breakthrough in the high-end bungee-based category, others have finally found a way to bring the price down to a much more affordable level.[39] With the equipment cost much less of a barrier for anyone interested in a serious fitness alternative—all you basically need is some light hand weights and to replace your bungee bands or springs eventually—we can look forward to the rapid growth of rebound exercise, possibly including Peloton- or MIRROR-like interfaces to facilitate group class and goal-oriented experiences.

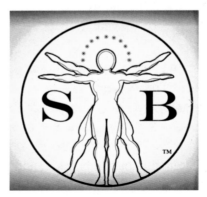

---

39 As we readily acknowledge, not everyone prefers bungee-based rebounders—for example, pronators can have problems, and runners may prefer mats supported with stiffer springs. Moreover, there are indeed some very high-quality spring-based rebounders still on the market. Nonetheless, most people we discuss this with acknowledge the overall superiority of the experience consistently delivered by high-quality bungee-based units.

Problems with Older Terminology for Bounce Types

Rebounders and rebound exercise go back to the mid-1970s. A partic-ular set of terminology that came into use at that time is still being used in most books, websites, and instructional materials on bouncing. This terminology, introduced primarily by the "father" of rebound exercise, Al Carter, categorizes bounces into five main types:

(1) Health bounces; (2) Aerobic bounces; (3) Strength bounces; (4) Sitting bounces; and (5) Assisted bounces.

As traditionally used, a "health bounce" is one in which some or all of your feet remain in contact with the mat as you bounce. The thinking goes something like this: even with little exertion, if someone is on the rebounder and moving at all—even with a very gentle up-and-down motion, with the feet remaining in one place and not leaving the mat at all—that individual will still receive at least some of the benefits of rebounding, including perhaps most importantly increased lymphatic circulation (which boosts immune system functioning).

A "health bounce" thus defined can easily be done by almost anyone (including those who need or prefer to use a stabilizer bar or other balance-assistance measures). The health bounce, then, was seemingly initially conceived of both as a warm-up exercise before more intensive rebounding as well as an end in and of itself, since it provides increased lymph flow, a cardiovascular training effect, and at least a minor effect on other body systems (e.g., the vestibular or inner ear system, the body's proprioceptive mechanisms, muscle tone and flexibility, and so on).

Next came the "aerobic bounce." Walking fast, running in place (all the way up to sprinting in place), dance steps, kicks, and so on were all considered aerobic bounces. The point here, of course, was to get one's heart rate up (to a safe range) and to work the cardiovascular system. Anything that moved the body fast enough was considered an aerobic bounce.

The third category was the "strength bounce." Here, the idea was to bounce as high as possible, or at least significantly up from the mat. According to Al Carter, "This is called the Strength Bounce because the vertical loading of acceleration, deceleration and gravity creates an increase in the G-force to which each cell of the body has to adjust. The higher the bounce, the greater the G-force."[40]

The fourth category was the "sitting bounce," which just as easily could have been named the "abdominal bounce." Fifth and last came "assisted bounces," such as the "Buddy Bounce" or a bounce using a bounce-back chair—that is, ways of using a rebounder for disabled folk who—with the help of a friend or the use of a special kind of rebounder—can still have a bit of the Bounce in their lives.

Problems with Traditional Terminology

The main thrust of how bounces were categorized was found in the first three of these categories: the health bounce, the aerobic bounce, and the strength bounce. There are two significant problems with this traditional terminology.

---

40 The equation of bouncing high with an increase in "cellular strength" due to increases in g-force is an interesting and provocative claim, but one that remains speculative. While it may be true—and would be a wonderful icing on the cake of the Bounce's many other benefits—it's not needed to explain why rebounding both feels so good and is so good for the human body.

First, it just does not give enough granularity or contain sufficient descriptive and explanatory power. Put simply, breaking everything down into three main categories is simply not sufficient, nor is it as useful as the system we use in chapter 5, "An Illustrated Compendium of Bounce Types and Movements."

Second, and perhaps more important, each of these terms is inherently somewhat misleading. For example, since *any* type of movement on a rebounder gives you increased lymph flow, it would be fairer to say that *all* bounces are health bounces, not just those that are very slow and mellow, and always keep the feet at least partly on the mat.

Similarly, since nearly all bouncing provides aerobic conditioning, and since most types of bounce movements can be done at any speed from very slowly to very rapidly and intensely, the term "aerobic bounce" is ultimately applicable to a wide variety of bouncing movements. Put differently, you can turn nearly any bounce into an aerobic bounce if you increase your speed and intensity, i.e., by moving into a higher "gear" as described at the end of Chapter 5.

Finally, equating high bounces with strength merely serves to lock in the unproven assumption about increased g-force—that more gravity exerts additional stress on all of your cells, so that all of you is cellularly strengthened—as to why bouncing is good for the human body. Instead, nearly all bounces increase your strength, especially if strength is defined in terms of both physical strength and flexibility. A simple example: if you use light hand weights to do resistive bouncing, you will both build up muscle and increase your flexibility, but you can do this without your feet ever leaving the mat. In this case, no high bouncing at all is necessary to increase your strength or tone and build muscle.

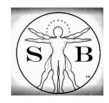

Notes

Here are some blank pages to record notes and observations. You can write about your:

- Favorite Bounce Types, movements, and routines
- Favorite music to bounce to
- Favorite friends and relatives to speak to while bouncing
- Amazing thoughts, ideas, feelings, and plans of action you have while bouncing, and whatever else comes across your mind before, during, or after the Bounce

It's *your space,* so please use it however you like! Write on!

The Bounce

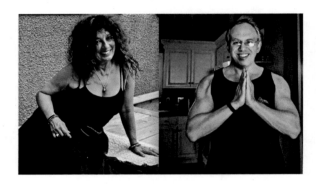

Joy Daniels and Jordan Gruber

The Bounce is the definitive new guidebook to rebound exercise, written by two devoted practitioners committed to sharing its transformative qualities.

Bouncing uniquely challenges and leverages gravity to safely but powerfully work your muscles (especially your core) while simultaneously providing aerobic conditioning and balance enhancement. By stimulating lymph flow, rebounding also enhances the immune system—something we can all benefit from—while reducing stress and enhancing psychological wellness and even spiritual practice.

Rebound exercise is fun (especially with music) and is well suited for home. This guidebook provides everything you need to know to successfully start, establish, and enjoy your own rebounding practice and the many benefits it can bring.

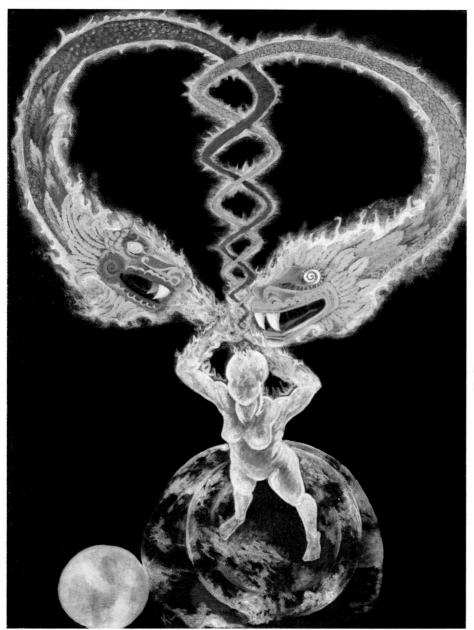

"Twin Dragons" by Krisztina Lazar